THE GUIDED IMAGERY HANDBOOK

THE GUIDED IMAGERY HANDBOOK

52 Scripts for Discovery & Recovery Using Symbols & Metaphor

for Therapists, Spiritual Practitioners & Self-Healers

KATHE CALDWELL, CCHT, G.I.T., CADC-II

CONTENTS

DEDICATION

To my loving husband, Tim, who always supports my endeavors and tells me, "It will be okay," just like I've asked him to. In all seriousness, he's the *best* friend and husband I could ever ask for!

And to my present and future clients and students, who continuously teach me about life, resilience, and the strength of the human spirit.

A NOTE FROM THE AUTHOR

PURPOSE

My purpose in writing this book is to introduce you to the simplicity, depth, and power of symbolic imagery. It is a fascinating and effective technique that can assist you to help others and yourself. My intention is for this book to be easy, functional, and experiential.

Through the years, my students and clients from my private practice and drug and alcohol programs have asked where they can find the imagery scripts I use. To my knowledge, there are few symbolic imageries that now exist in this particular script version with corresponding questions. I began writing and collecting them in 2002.

In fact, I didn't learn imagery with scripts, and I like to teach imagery without them. I do, however, understand how valuable these scripts can be when doing individual or group work and how they fill in the gap between passive and interactive imagery.

As I've continued to write and gather imagery through the years, creating a book for others' benefit came naturally. Imagery changed my life, and I know what an amazing gift it can be for people in transition, recovery, and those wanting an effective self-inquiry tool.

This is why I bring this book into the world . . . for you.

IMAGERY USING SYMBOLS AND METAPHOR

Although all imagery is metaphoric and symbolic by nature, I'm identifying the imageries in this book as symbolic imagery because the symbols are the *primary* focus and method through which the participant receives meaning.

Each imagery experience is unique to each individual. I have given you suggestions and examples along the way to help you become comfortable in asking the right questions to bring understanding to the participant.

PASSIVE IMAGERY FOR INDIVIDUALS AND GROUPS

This book is an introduction to symbolic imagery. The scripts are designed to be read to individuals or groups, who passively listen as they experience the imagery. After the imagery, the questions are answered, verbally and/or written, and then discussed. For information on learning more about the therapeutic technique of Guided Imagery, see Chapter 7 (Resources).

USE OF THE TERMS *PRACTITIONER* AND *PARTICIPANT*

Individual, counselor, therapist, or group facilitator = **Practitioner**

Person experiencing the imagery = **Participant**

Imagery can be used in many therapeutic environments: medical, psychotherapy, physical therapy, hypnotherapy, drug and alcohol treatment, sound therapy, spiritual, secular, reiki, self-healing, etc. For ease of use, I have termed the facilitator (reader of the imagery) as *practitioner* and the person(s) experiencing the imagery as *participant*.

I have also identified unspecified singular beings, persons, or animals seen in imagery or within a group as **they/them/their**.

SUBCONSCIOUS VS. UNCONSCIOUS

The words *subconscious* and *unconscious* are often used interchangeably, though there is a difference between the two. Being a hypnotherapist, I prefer to use the word **subconscious** instead of the word *unconscious*. *Unconscious* can refer to both the "deeper mind" and to those things that are unknown that affect our beliefs and behavior; it can also refer to the state of *being* unconscious. The French psychologist Pierre Janet coined the term *subconscious*, which refers to those things that are not conscious at the moment but are possible to be recalled. When I use the word *subconscious*, I am referring to this definition.

REPETITION

As a teacher, I know the importance of repetition in learning. I have repeated the following facts throughout this book to empower you and the participant to trust, respect, and relax into the process of imagery:

FOUR IMPORTANT FACTS ★★★★

1. *Allow* whatever comes up in imagery to be. It is more about discovery than concrete answers. Imagery has more to do with the heart and soul; to feelings and intuition, than the intellect.
2. There is no right or wrong in imagery. People experience what they're meant to experience, courtesy of their own imaginations.
3. Personal symbols are most important for the participant. You aren't responsible for giving them the meaning. The right questions, conversation, and time will organically elicit understanding.
4. Some of the subjects addressed can be poignant. Respect the participants' belief systems, responses, and feelings. Again . . . *allow*.

INTRODUCTION
GUIDED TO IMAGERY

When my best friend and I were in our twenties, we would regularly shout out, "It's a sign! It's a sign!" when something important happened. Sometimes we were serious, and other times it was silliness; but I have always believed in signs. That was why, at my lowest point, I asked for a sign that guided me to imagery.

When I first discovered symbolic imagery twenty years ago, I was going through one of the hardest times in my life.

Several years earlier, I had noticed that I was always out of energy and needed twice the sleep. One morning, I felt as though I'd developed arthritis overnight. Instead of feeling like a healthy forty-eight-year-old, I felt like an unhealthy eighty-year-old.

My job doing administrative work for an international manufacturing company became almost impossible. Going to bed by seven most nights barely allowed my body to function during the day. Fate intervened when my company returned to Japan, and I was unemployed. But despite not working, my body continued to weaken. I couldn't eat and lost twenty pounds in a short amount of time. I weighed what I had at twelve years old. Often, my husband had to help me to the bathroom.

Something was wrong, and no test could name it.

For a year, I saw numerous allopathic and holistic doctors. One psychologist kindly charged me less to help me deal with my "new normal," which wasn't normal at all. I couldn't work in this condition. For twenty years, I had worked primarily in administration, with some alcohol and drug counseling weaved in. Now, I couldn't even handle that amount of physical activity. Worst of all, I didn't know who I was anymore.

How would I survive?

Sleep was often hard to come by. On my lowest night, I lay awake trying to read a book. Holding it open with my hands hurt too much, so I had an object propping the book up against my husband's pillow. Each page I turned brought me to tears.

In desperation, I said, "God, if I'm going to die, so be it! But If I'm not, and I have a purpose to complete, please give me a sign! I need a reason. I'll do whatever I'm supposed to do, but I need a sign!"

After giving up on reading, a song ran through my mind that I'd heard at a church years earlier. While I had never participated much in organized religion, I believed strongly in my own spiritual connection to God. The song is titled, "It's in Every One of Us."

It's in every one of us to be wise,
Find your heart
Open up both your eyes,
We can all know everything
Without ever knowing why,
It's in every one of us
By and by [1]

That song wouldn't stop! It played over and over in my mind, like a looped TV jingle I couldn't turn off. *Why this song?* I thought. As it continued, it just added to my frustration and exhaustion.

When the sun burst through our bedroom window that morning, I realized that maybe this was the sign I had asked for. Maybe the song was directing me to go back to that church? That's when I also realized it was Sunday morning!

After getting out of bed, I had one hope: that there was something at that church that would give me another sign.

Fifty people filled the congregation when my mother and I sat down. The choir sang a current, rhythmic, inspirational song, and I cried from beginning to end. All the frustration and fear I'd been holding back for a year suddenly broke open and poured out of me.

After my emotional release, I regained my composure and wiped the last of my tears away. I felt like an empty barrel with the wind blowing through me—raw and open. I announced to my mother, "I'm joining that choir. I can sing once a week." This one thing I knew I could do.

And just this one thing brought me hope.

The next week, I sat in a chair at choir practice. Singing was the perfect outlet for me. It didn't increase pain and distracted me from it. During a break, everyone left the stage, and only one woman remained sitting near me. Having nothing to do, I asked her, "What's your name?"

"Teri," she said.
"I'm Kathe. What do you do?"
"I'm a guided imagery therapist."

This intrigued me! She had my full attention. I knew guided imagery. But a guided imagery *therapist?*

Once she'd explained how she used guided imagery, I said, "I've done that all my life! I help my family and friends interpret their dreams. *I* can do that! Where do I begin?"

She directed me to Dr. Charles Leviton who taught at a local college.

A friend had given me a late enrollment form that needed to be signed by the college chancellor. When I arrived at the college, the huge parking lot was packed, and I was forced to park at the outer edges. It was the beginning of a long walk. After

1   by David Pomeranz

a few steps out of the car, I could feel that my body had already "hit the wall." When that happened, it felt like my life force had been sucked out of every cell. It was frightening, as though I had to overpower my body with my mind to make it work.

Once I'd started walking toward the college, there was no turning back. I counted my steps— sometimes I'd make it to twenty before I'd have to sit down, cross-legged, on the asphalt. I didn't care what people thought; I was headed toward the chancellor's office, and I was going to get into the Guided Imagery class! Several people asked me if I was okay as I sat on the asphalt in the midst of hundreds of cars. I'd say, "Yeah, just resting my back," and eventually get up and carry on. Twenty steps, fifteen, and sometimes ten at a time.

Finally, I reached the right building, got into the chancellor's office, and dropped my body into the first chair I saw. When I had regained enough energy, I got up and asked his assistant to see the chancellor. She walked me to his desk and gestured for me to sit. The chancellor looked like he was in his sixties and having a very bad day.

I handed him my form and politely told him, "I need your signature to get into class."

He said, "I can't do it, it's too late" and handed the form back to me without looking at me.

I explained that I hadn't worked in over a year and needed this class.

He repeated, "Can't do it."

I said, "I can't work at anything even slightly physical; I need a new career, *and I think this is it!*"

He stared at me, unimpressed.

I tried again, "I know it's nothing to you. It's just a signature. But to me, it's my life! And if I don't have this, I don't have hope. *Please!*"

"It's against the rules." His face was expressionless.

I felt my lower lip start to quiver. A wave of emotion welled up within me, and I felt the warmth of tears fill my eyes. I was six years old again, powerless to hide my disappointment. Even I hadn't realized how important this was. I couldn't hold the tears back.

The chancellor looked everywhere but at me and then stared down at his desk. His assistant appeared again and grabbed the form from my hand, and I thought, *It's over.* She then held it under her boss's face. "Just sign it! Sign it!" she said.

He sat motionless, still looking downward. Silence.

Again, more softly, she urged, *"Just sign it."*

Time slowed down as I stared at him, my vision blurred by tears. Excruciating silence.

Then, he was reaching for his pen. With his head still lowered, he said, "Don't ever tell anyone I did this!"

(Thank you, Chancellor! You changed someone's life for the better, just by signing your name!)

The next week, I sat in class, thrilled to be in the world with a purpose and a goal.

In time, I was diagnosed with fibromyalgia, which I didn't think fit, though I had some of the symptoms. I continued to improve over time, regaining the ability to eat normally. The pain would come and go, with some good days and plenty of bad days. Meanwhile, I began learning everything I could about guided imagery as well as hypnosis, attending Dr. Leviton's class and training at the Academy for Guided Imagery and American Pacific University.

Eventually, I began working for drug and alcohol rehabilitation centers doing both imagery and hypnosis. Adding hypnosis and imagery complemented the drug and alcohol counseling I had started years earlier. Most importantly, it was wonderfully soothing and insightful for clients.

Using these mind-body methods also gave me the calmness that I hadn't felt when doing straight talk-therapy years before. Slowly, I began to develop my own style. Over and over I witnessed just how beneficial imagery was for clients. I opened my own private practice and later began teaching.

It wasn't until I was completely settled into a career in hypnosis and guided imagery that I found the true source of my pain and weakness: I had toxic metals in my body. If I had found out prior to that time, I might have gone back into the corporate sector. I was relieved to finally know the cause of my health issues, and I began therapy to heal my body.

The truth is, my journey happened in the perfect time to allow me to fulfill my purpose and the pact I'd made with God years before. There had been a bigger plan for me than I could have imagined. When I asked for help, followed the signs, and took action, I was given everything I needed to *live* my purpose.

We all go through personal life challenges and transitions. I hope that this book will be useful to you in following the signs on your own journey and helping others on theirs. And if you are going through a life challenge now, I wish you hope, courage, and the message to *not give up!* We're all here to help one another, which is my intention for this book.

I hope you enjoy exploring the amazing landscape of the subconscious mind. The journey into ourselves can be the most fascinating and important journey we ever take.

CHAPTER 1
WHAT IS GUIDED IMAGERY?

"The soul never thinks without a picture." ~Aristotle

"Imagination is the language of the soul. Pay attention to your imagination
and you will discover all you need to be fulfilled." ~Albert Einstein

DEFINITION OF GUIDED IMAGERY

The two simplest definitions of guided imagery that I like are:

1. Purposefully utilizing the five senses within the imagination (to see, hear, touch, feel, smell and sense) toward a goal.
2. Being intentionally guided by another person into your imagination for a purpose. (Some examples: self-discovery, stress reduction, relaxation, physical or emotional healing, spiritual connection, empowerment, motivation, and performance.)

WE ARE ALL IMAGINING ALL THE TIME

Brain imaging studies using fMRI at the University of Colorado at Boulder and Icahn School of Medicine[2] confirmed that our brains do not know the difference between imagining something or actually experiencing it.

From the time we awaken, we begin to imagine. In order to even get out of bed, we have to *imagine* it happening—sometimes several times in a row on a lazy morning!

We imagine our day ahead. We imagine future conversations and past conversations we *wish* we'd had. We imagine tasks to complete. We imagine attaining desires and goals, careers, and life partners. We imagine every day from morning till night.

Everything that has ever been created by humans first started with imagination. Why not go exploring in our imaginal landscape to discover more about ourselves? There are infinite possibilities within this creative universe. And because we are all imagining all the time, and the mind doesn't know the difference between what's "real" and "what's imagined," then why not use the imagination to focus on what we truly desire?

2 ScienceDaily.com, Science News, December 10, 2018

SYMBOLIC IMAGERY

This book focuses on symbolic therapeutic imagery. This imagery allows the discovery of deeper parts of ourselves through seeing symbols. The practitioner guides the participant on a journey into the participant's imagination, allowing the participant's subconscious to bring up what is important.

The beauty of symbolic imagery is that it bypasses judgment, making it a wonderful tool to circumvent resistance and denial.

There is no right or wrong in imagery; it is simply informational. It is a gentle yet powerful tool to open up windows into ourselves to discover, release, and receive direction.

Through guided imagery, we can speak to our higher power or higher self, to our cells and physiological processes, to our loved ones, and even to our past and future selves. We can tap into our own guidance system, which may turn out to be a wizard, angel, spiritual being, animal, or a known or unknown person. Imagery can move you toward physical and emotional healing as well as bring insights that teach and inspire you.

As an introduction to symbolic guided imagery, this book provides just a portion of what one can do with imagery. There are many types of imagery and different ways to facilitate it. If you are a seasoned practitioner, you can modify the imageries in this book for interactive imagery, which goes beyond the scope of this book.

Because we can go anywhere in our imaginations, imagery gives us the ability to release old beliefs from the past that no longer benefit us or to visualize future success and happiness.

We can stretch our imaginations toward new beliefs, new behavior, and improved performance. We can invite wise and loving guides to join us on our journey. We can have conversations with loved ones who have passed or loved ones we hope to know in the future. There are endless possibilities for guided imagery's uses. It can physically and emotionally calm us, advise us, help us tap into our intuitions and creativity, increase self-awareness and confidence, boost our immune systems, and connect us with our spirituality.

TYPES OF IMAGERY

#	TYPE OF IMAGERY	PURPOSE	AN EXAMPLE
1	**Cellular**	Imagining and directing specific cells toward a desired healthy outcome. (Must research cell's behavior)	Imagining immune cells surrounding and attacking cancer cells.
2	**End-state**	Imagining yourself in the state you desire: Examples: healthy, at peace, confident, successful, etc.	Imagining yourself standing in front of a crowd, speaking easily and confidently. You're calm and focused, and enjoy sharing your knowledge with others.
3	**Energetic**	To rebalance and unlock the body's energy flow (prana/ chi).	Imagining/feeling the vibrational energy flowing freely through your body. Often used with sound, breath and body therapies.
4	**Feeling-state**	Changing one's feeling-state from one emotion to another.	Imagining a soothing, peaceful scene or whatever changes an anxious state to a calm state.
5	**Metaphoric (Symbolic)**	Receive information from the deeper self to inform, heal, inspire, motivate, etc.	Imagining a symbol of your fear (and possibly dialoguing with it) to discover, understand, and transform it.
6	**Physiological**	Imagining physiological changes in the body required for greater health. (Research required to know proper physical mechanics of body)	Imagining your blood pressure naturally decreasing as your arteries widen and become more flexible.
7	**Psychological**	To shift our perception of ourselves, and our emotional challenges.	Imagining your anger as a place in your body and having a conversation with it.
8	**Spiritual**	Connecting to one's faith and spirituality.	Imagining a representation of your faith and spirituality appearing in a form your subconscious creates.

*Author's Note:

- This book focuses on symbolic imagery, highlighted above, though many of the types of imagery can coexist within one imagery.

- Table compiled from Belleruth Naparstek's book *Staying Well With Guided Imagery*

HOW IT FEELS: USING OUR FIVE SENSES WITHIN THE IMAGINATION

Experiencing guided imagery is like being taken through a "waking dream" using our five senses. Let's say you're guided to the beach within your imagination. Depending on your primary mode of sensory intake, you might *see* the calm waves coming in, *feel* the breeze on your skin, *hear* the palm trees rustling, *smell* the scent of the ocean, or even *taste* the salt from the water. You might simply *sense* the peacefulness and tranquility and experience the emotion of contentment.

Guided imagery is extremely relaxing. I often explain it as that feeling right before you go to sleep: your breathing becomes rhythmic and you know where you are, but you're too content to care. Many people don't want imagery to end, because they're enjoying the experience so much.

Imagery works through the subconscious and your parasympathetic nervous system. As you calm your body with imagery, your heart rate and blood pressure slow. Breathing regulates, muscles relax, and the entire body receives rest and rejuvenation.

Both the practitioner and the participant receive benefits from this calming of the body-mind. The more the practitioner relaxes into the imagery as they read it, the deeper the participant can experience it. Being open and experiencing the participant as a partner in this creative journey is the very essence of imagery's effectiveness. Imagery is always about allowing, not forcing. I also find that the more open and permissive the language is, the better people respond to it.

EXAMPLES OF SYMBOLIC IMAGERY

Within symbolic imagery, we visualize symbols that represent emotions, situations, people, and abstract ideas. Once the symbol is present, a dialogue between the participant and the symbol can be initiated to receive information. All imagery is metaphoric and symbolic; however, therapeutic symbolic imagery uses symbols as the *primary* focus and method through which the participant receives meaning. No matter that a symbol might be inanimate; in the imagination, *everything is possible*.

See examples below of what a practitioner might say to a participant and what the participant may see:

Examples:

Book = Purpose (Situation)
"See a symbol that represents your goal."
The participant could see a book that represents learning/education.

Lightning Bolt = Anger (Emotion)
"See a symbol that represents your anger."
The participant could see a volcano, lightning bolt, etc.

Lion = Parent (Person)
"See an animal that represents your father."
The participant could see a lion or an eagle that can give them a message through feelings and/or words.

Metaphoric symbolic imagery is the most commonly used guided imagery. Metaphoric imagery uses one thing to symbolize another: such as a storm representing challenges and a fence representing boundaries.

Examples:

<u>Storm = Challenges</u>
"The storm (challenges) began to lessen and patches of blue sky appeared."

<u>Fence = Boundaries</u>
"The fence (boundary) fell and the horse realized it could run free."

WAKING DREAMS

In imagery, we access the subconscious mind just as we do while dreaming.

Imagery is a type of "waking dream" created for specific purposes. In imagery, as in visions and dreams, seeing symbols allows us to delve deeper into understanding our beliefs, emotions, and behavior. Our subconscious mind creates symbols that represent our emotions.

Have you ever had a dream that left you with a feeling that stayed with you all day or even several days? Those dreams, like imagery, can hold important messages. Dreams can also act as a release of feelings we have suppressed or were unaware of. The meaning of the imagery or dream is derived from interpreting the symbols.

GUIDED IMAGERY IS SIMILAR TO DREAMING WHILE IN A RELAXED, WAKING STATE

The importance of receiving messages through dreams is referenced throughout history. Over twenty dreams and innumerable visions are referenced in the Christian Bible and Hebrew scriptures. Some come as warnings, some as clarification, and some for spiritual direction. A vision happens while you are awake, and a dream occurs while you are unconscious.[3]

The Navajo tribe encourages dreamers to verbalize their dreams with a trusted family member as soon as possible after awakening. Irene Yazzie claims that, ". . . dreams cannot be kept inside: You have to talk about it. I mean verbalize it [and] try to figure out what it is trying to say." [4]

The Senoi people, an indigenous tribe in Malaysia, spend time each and every day recalling and sharing their dreams with one another. Tribe members learn to face their fears while dreaming, to move toward pleasure, and to do their best to change their dreams toward success.[5]

There is a tribe in Ecuador that dreams collectively with the intention of accessing information for the entire tribe to act upon.

Guided imagery affords us the opportunity to receive this guidance in a relaxed, waking state.

---

3   Quora.com, difference between vision and dream.
4   Three Diné Women on the Navajo Approach to Dreams, John Dadosky
5   How the Remote Senoi Tribes Use Dreams for Personal Growth, Victoria G. Duda, Ph.D.

GUIDED IMAGERY BY ANY OTHER NAME

Some of the terms you may see used interchangeably to describe guided imagery are as follows:

- Active Imagination
- Creative Visualization
- Guided Affective Imagery
- Guided Meditation
- Guided Mental Imagery
- Intentional Imagining
- Mental Imagery
- Visualization

Though these terms were created by persons using imagery in their own particular way, all of the terms fall under the definition of "imagining on purpose, for a purpose." However, "Guided Imagery" refers to using *all* of the senses, not only visual.

CHAPTER 2
BENEFITS OF GUIDED IMAGERY

Guided imagery has *innumerable* benefits because it is holistic: inclusive of mind, body, and spirit. When we connect with the imagination—or the subconscious— we can affect positive changes in the *whole* person. Each of the 52 imageries within this book can be used as easy, structured therapy within an hour.

Guided imagery can create simple relaxation, improve performance, and advance physical and emotional healing, self-discovery, creativity, inspiration, and empowerment. And don't forget *fun!* I often get the pleasure of seeing a wide smile come over a client's face as they reconnect with their childhood innocence and wonder, see someone important from their past, or burst into peals of laughter from envisioning something unexpected.

HOW SYMBOLIC IMAGERY BRINGS AWARENESS

Communing with nature, animals, objects, spiritual beings, or people from the imaginal mind allows participants to learn from the images (symbols) they see and dialogue with. No matter how difficult the truth they receive, there is no one to "blame" because the information arises from their own subconscious. And because symbols are visual representations created from our own beliefs and emotions, symbols elicit very personal insights. Once information has come up to our conscious awareness, we then have the ability to address it. Imagery is gentle yet powerful—it can bring layers of understanding and emergent meaning to those who experience it.

Deeper meaning from imagery can continue to surface as time goes on. Clients have told me that they suddenly understood more profound aspects of an imagery's meaning one or two years after experiencing it. I myself have personally experienced this. I often call imagery "the gift that keeps on giving."

Who doesn't like that?

BENEFITS IN DISCOVERY AND RECOVERY

I have worked with people in substance abuse recovery for many years, and I love it. I love seeing the light come back into people's eyes. I love seeing the "real" person come out from under the veil of addiction. Some of the most wonderful people I've ever met have had the disease of addiction. And I've witnessed how powerful symbolic imagery can be for those in recovery. It allows relief from anxiety, overthinking, and the judgment of the conscious mind. Clients can relax in the knowledge that there is no right or wrong in it, even as they access consequential self-exploration and greater self-awareness.

The "rehab weary" often get tired of being told what to do and when to do it. As necessary as rigorous rules and regulations are, I'm often told that it's a joy to receive direction from their own inner wisdom for a change! There can also be a profound depth to the feeling of the imagery that stays with the participant as, or until, emerging truth is realized, as often happens with dreaming. And because imagery doesn't lie, the inner direction received is hard to dispute.

Receiving valuable information and insight from one's own inner wisdom can also be empowering. There's often a reconnection with spirituality through symbols and metaphor, which can be unexpected, perception-changing, and even transformational.

The truth is simply the truth. They are communicating, or communing, with their own spirit and their own connection to their personal source of faith.

USE OF SYMBOLS ENCOURAGES OPENNESS AND VULNERABILITY

What is discussed through explaining imagery is not intellectual; it is feeling-based and somatic. Participants are able to express greater vulnerability and openness as their feelings come through symbols and metaphor.

Clients can have deep conversations with cartoon characters. They can laugh and cry with their deceased grandparent. They can give support to their inner child or receive inspiration and information from their future self. They can receive valuable information from inanimate objects like a car, backpack, or a giant marshmallow heart.

People enjoy sharing what their imagination has created. Seeing animals, objects, wizards, people known and unknown, and spiritual beings can bring revelations, tears of joy, and sometimes childlike laughter. And because it is generated from their subconscious, it is highly individual and relevant to their life at present.

Whether working with individuals or groups, imagery assists clients to:

- Connect with the authentic self
- Have fun through the imagination
- Promote thought-provoking questions
- Arrive at refreshing new concepts or ideas
- Laugh to release physical stress

FOCUS AND BENEFITS OF THE 52 IMAGERIES

- Acceptance / Allowance / Trust
- Addiction / Sobriety
- Being Present
- Childhood / Inner Child
- Clarity
- Confidence
- Faith / Spirituality
- Forgiveness

- Grief / Sadness
- Health / Well-being
- Inspiration / Motivation
- Relationships
- Release
- Self-Awareness / Self-Discovery
- Self-Care / Self Love

IMAGERY'S EMOTIONAL BENEFITS

- Offers discovery and direction from one's own inner wisdom
- Bypasses denial and resistance by using symbols and metaphor
- Allows self-participation in healing
- Can release emotional pain
- Allows one to connect and converse with past, future, or current loved ones
- Can release and ease grief
- Can reframe past experiences for healing
- Can work toward forgiveness
- Assists to confirm feelings, beliefs, and progress
- Proposes new perspectives
- Inspires self-love, self-esteem, and integration
- Presents new possibilities by experiencing them as real through the five senses in the imagination

Example: Grandfather = Love

Message = "Keep going"

Hayden has been having difficulty with guilt and shame due to previous substance use. He sees his grandfather in an imagery and says that his grandfather represents love to him. He explains that his grandfather died three years ago. His grandfather loved him completely and wanted only happiness for him.

Within the imagery, his grandfather puts his hands on Hayden's shoulders, looks into his eyes, and says, "You're worth it, Hayden! I'm with you every day. Keep going!"

Hayden's eyes well up with tears as he explains the experience. He says, "Everything about my grandfather was good, and that's what he saw in me. I want to make him proud." Hayden later says that he remembers this experience when things get difficult and he needs encouragement.

Example: Jesus = Peace, Love, Comfort

Leticia is surprised to have Jesus appear in her imagery. She explains, "I haven't been into religion since I was a kid." Within the imagery, Leticia feels the unconditional love and peace of Jesus. Since she's been feeling lonely, it brings tears to her eyes and she tells the group, "I felt so loved and comforted. Jesus said, 'Remember, you're never alone.'"

IMAGERY'S SPIRITUAL BENEFITS

In my private practice, when I ask clients to invite an inner guide for spiritual guidance, they visualize angels, bodies of light, God, ancestors, goddesses, shamans, the Divine Mother, Jesus, alchemists, and other beings. Whoever brings the message, it is just the right message that brings grace, inspiration, and whatever that individual needs.

The Recovery Research Institute, a nonprofit institution of Massachusetts General Hospital (an affiliate of Harvard Medical School), is conducting brain imaging studies on spirituality. Many approaches to recovery, such as mindfulness-based therapies, incorporate spiritual practices without a request to believe in higher power or religion.

They found that spirituality was associated with reduced activity in the medial thalamus and striatum, brain regions implicated in sensory and emotional processing, indicating that spirituality may help us focus and control our emotions.[6]

Though science continues working to prove what might only be able to be felt and experienced through the human spirit, I say more power to scientific research! Each person comes to their own spiritual connection in different ways, and more roads leading to that connection make it more accessible to all—and that's a gift. I believe that spirituality *is* the basis of guided imagery and other experiential modalities, but whether it is called science or spirituality, it is the positive change that is key in therapy. There is a beauty, simplicity, and power of connecting with that which is greater than ourselves, whatever you choose to call it. Whatever the religious, spiritual, or secular beliefs of my clients, they often have profound experiences during imagery that are remembered for years which inspire and comfort them.

> **Example:** God = Unconditional Love
> Heart = Gift
> Key = New Life

Tiffany visualizes an older woman with long white hair and the kindest eyes she's ever seen, who she says represents God. Tiffany says she feels unconditional love emanating from her. She smiles through tears. She explains that she doesn't believe in a higher power, so she is surprised at her vision. She then describes seeing a glowing pink heart in her hands, which she hands to the woman who represents God. In return, the woman gives her a key, which she says is the key to her new life.

> **Example:** Sage = Love
> Message = "Stay connected"

Within her imagery, Maribel sees a sage who says his name is Yaro. Yaro has deep, twinkling brown eyes. Maribel feels his love and support. Yaro gives her the message, "Keep meditating and stay connected to your higher power."

---

6   www.recoveryanswers.org/research-post/spirituality-brain-imagining-addiction/

PHYSICAL BENEFITS

- Lowers stress, heart rate and blood pressure
- Decreases anxiety and calms the parasympathetic nervous system
- Creates whole brain activity, optimizing mental and emotional health
- Sends healing chemicals throughout the body
- Boosts the immune system
- Can reduce pain and the sensation of pain
- Improves surgery/medical outcomes

Example: Emotional and Physical Calming

Years ago, I was visiting a friend in the hospital, doing imagery with her as her nurse administered her therapy. After I said goodbye to my friend and began walking down the corridor, her nurse ran after me, tapped me on the shoulder, and asked, "Could you follow me around the hospital today?"

She explained that she'd never seen a patient calm down that much while receiving treatment. Of course, I couldn't follow her around the hospital that day, but many nurses and others in the healthcare field have learned guided imagery for that particular reason. They find imagery an amazingly effective tool to emotionally and physically empower their patients.

If guided imagery can calm patients in the hospital, it can certainly relax clients in a therapy office, recovery setting, or anywhere else. I have used it on myself in medical settings when I needed courage and reassurance. Being able to call on an inner guide is a wonderful self-soothing tool for self-support.

HOSPITALS' USE OF GUIDED IMAGERY FOR PATIENTS

In 1996, Henry Bennett and Henry Dreher researched 335 surgery patients at UC Davis School of Medicine in a randomized, placebo-controlled, double-blind clinical study (completed at Penn State). Before surgery, they gave four groups one of the following: affirmation tapes, hemi-sync sound tapes, guided imagery tapes, or nothing (for the control group).

The guided imagery group lost 50 percent less blood in surgery, had less stress, shorter hospital stays, and faster healing. The hospital saved over $2,000 per patient. [7]

"More than 200 research studies in the past thirty years have explored the role of mind-body techniques in helping people prepare for surgical and medical procedures and in helping them recover more rapidly. These studies show that guided imagery can dramatically counteract a loss of control, fear, panic, anxiety, helplessness and uncertainty." [8]

Due to the financial viability, many hospitals now utilize guided imagery recordings for surgery preparation. For more information on imagery for health and wellness, see books listed in Chapter 7 (Resources) by Belleruth Naparstek and Dr. Marty Rossman. Belleruth Naparstek's website www.healthjourneys has hundreds of audio recordings available for physical, emotional, and spiritual healing.

---

7   Advances in Mind-Body Medicine, Interviews for Surgery: Evidence and Exigency."
8   Myclevelandclinic.org/departments/wellness/integrative/treatments-service/guidedimagery#research

CHAPTER 3
HOW TO USE THE IMAGERIES

FOUR IMPORTANT FACTS ★★★★

1. *Allow* whatever comes up in imagery to be. It is more about discovery than concrete answers. Imagery has more to do with the heart and soul; to feelings and intuition, than the intellect.
2. There is no right or wrong in imagery. People experience what they're meant to experience, courtesy of their own imaginations.
3. Personal symbols are most important for the participant. You aren't responsible for giving them the meaning. The right questions, conversation, and time will organically elicit understanding.
4. Some of the subjects addressed can be poignant. Respect the participants' belief systems, responses, and feelings. Again . . . *allow*.

The imagery scripts in this book are intentionally written in an open, simple style to allow participants to visualize what is most relevant and important to them. Each imagery is intended to be read to an individual or group.

Before reading the imagery, let the participant(s) know that there is no right or wrong in imagery. Whatever is most important will arise from their subconscious minds.

Do not tell the participant(s) what the imagery represents until after they have experienced it and shared it with you. This allows them to release judgment from the conscious mind of what they think they should see.

An exception to this rule: If you are a practitioner working with a client who has experienced trauma, and feel the imagery could be sensitive material for them, then discuss the subject matter with the client to decide whether to utilize it or not.

And because the imagination is limitlessly creative and individual, participants will sometimes see a desert although the practitioner described the ocean. Whatever is seen is pertinent for the individual.

Let participants know that symbolic imagery is not just exploratory, it can be fun, fascinating, and sometimes even funny. They can relax while listening. You can also enjoy the process and relax into spontaneity—that is the key to discovery.

A CALM, SAFE, CONFIDENTIAL ENVIRONMENT

- Let the participant(s) know that they're in a safe space where they can express themselves freely and confidentially.
- Clarify that there is no right or wrong in the imagination! Whatever they visualize is what is important.

- The environment should be free of strong scents, bright lights, pets, or people that might interrupt.
- Turn off all phones.
- Although a quiet space is the optimal environment for imagery, I have guided individuals or groups through imagery in some noisy situations. It didn't stop participant(s) from having good experiences. There are some people who are noise sensitive, but we do the best we can! In those situations, I tell clients that going inward and letting go of outside noise is good practice for meditation and mindfulness.

MUSIC

- Music is not a necessity, but it can be a wonderful and soothing complement to imagery. The right music can entrain one into, and continually deepen, relaxation. Very occasionally I'll have someone who does not want music, and I honor that, of course.
- I use instrumental, ambient music that is simple, calm, and meandering. Stay away from changing rhythms or cultural music that could interject specific scenes into the participant's mind. There is an abundance of relaxation music (new age, massage, meditation) available online to choose from.
- If doing imagery with sound therapy, you can of course choose what music/sounds complement the imagery and vice-versa.
- It's best to use longer tracks, at least ten to fifteen minutes long, for the set imageries.
- If you would like to add sound effects to a particular imagery, such as Rain, do so very sparingly and make sure the sounds are gentle and don't overpower the imagery.

Imagery evokes the imagination and five senses sufficiently without enhancement. I once heard about an enthusiastic imagery student who put her group of peers in a circle. They closed their eyes as she suggested, and she guided them in a lovely waterfall imagery. As they became extremely relaxed, she began spraying them with a water mister she thought would heighten the experience. It did!

Several students in the circle jumped out of their chairs screaming! You get the idea.

CHOOSING THE IMAGERY

The imageries are listed alphabetically, and then listed categorically by purpose in Chapter Five.

Important: Do not tell participant(s) the focus and meaning of the imagery that you have chosen. Let them experience it without having prior time to think about it or decide to visualize something in particular. The beauty of imagery is that it is spontaneous and *felt* or *sensed* rather than thought. In this regard, imagery doesn't lie. It knows us better than we know ourselves. Allow people to experience the imagery without forethought.

On my client intake form in my private practice, I ask whether clients have any fears or phobias. If I'm aware that a client has a fear of water, I obviously won't choose a water-related imagery, such as River.

I've done imagery work with groups and individuals for many years and found that it's rare to have negative, fearful experiences. This, of course, is different if you're working with a client or clients with trauma. If a participant is uncomfortable, they will normally just open their eyes and stop imagining. If they are uncomfortable closing their eyes, I tell them that is fine; we imagine with our eyes open all day, every day. I never press people to do imagery. It is not for everyone. Usually people with trauma enjoy imagery very much—and receive great benefit from it. It is a matter of them feeling safe within the relationship with the practitioner.

Choose an imagery which fits your participant's needs best *at present*.

If I find that an individual or group is weary from a hard day, I will choose a simpler imagery that veers toward relaxation rather than deeper exploration.

TIME ALLOTTED FOR IMAGERY

Group: Generally One Hour

Most of the imageries take from five to seven minutes to read. When I do a group of up to six people, it takes a full hour to discuss all of their imagery experiences. More than six people is difficult to do in a one-hour period. If you have more than six, give yourself more time if possible, or choose one of the shorter, simpler imageries, such as T-Shirt or Coat.

Individual: Thirty Minutes to One Hour

Working with an individual gives you time to ask more questions and delve more deeply into the imagery's symbols and meaning. You and the individual can gather insightful information and possible direction for future exploration. If the imagery and debriefing take only a half-hour, you can use the remaining time to discuss what was learned and how it can be used beneficially, or you can do another activity related to your purpose.

READING THE IMAGERIES

TO A GROUP OR INDIVIDUAL

- Reading the short relaxation portion of each imagery is adequate to relax participants. It takes as little as one to three minutes to become relaxed for symbolic imagery. And you can always choose to add a favorite relaxation/induction of your own.
- As soon as a person becomes engaged with their inner senses, they have separated from the critical, conscious mind and are in their imaginal mind.

USING YOUR VOICE AS A TOOL

Use your voice as a tool. Speak in a soft, yet clear, audible voice.

- Emphasize words that increase relaxation, such as *soothing, peaceful, relaxed,* etc.

- Read slowly and pause between questions to allow participants time to visually and emotionally process what they're experiencing in their inner world.
- Participants will entrain to the rhythm of your voice. They will respond as you slow down or pick up the pace. You are the channel through which imagery flows; your relaxed demeanor will initiate their relaxation.
- Bring participants back from the imagery slowly. Increase the volume and then the speed of your voice as you read. After they have opened their eyes, allow them at least five to ten seconds to refocus before asking questions or having them write answers to the questions from the Insight page.

RECORDING THE IMAGERY SESSION

If your individual client is interested in having the imagery session recorded, the easiest way is for the client to record it on their personal phone. If they aren't aware of how to do that, I show them, or record it on mine if they request that and then email or text it to them. Technology offers many choices now, and you can choose whatever technology best suits you and the level of professionalism you strive for.

LEARNING THROUGH EXPERIENCE

Symbolic imagery is an experiential tool. If you haven't experienced it yourself, the best way to understand it is to *experience* it. Choose a few imageries that resonate with you. Have a friend or colleague read the imagery to you and ask you the questions. Once you've experienced it yourself, you'll have a much better feel for the pacing, how to utilize your voice, and how to ask the questions. You'll also realize how beneficial it can be and how it feels to be on the listening and experiencing end as the participant.

TRUST THE SUBCONSCIOUS

The subconscious mind creates symbols that represent participants' *genuine* feelings and beliefs. It also offers guidance toward future direction, authenticity, and self-awareness.

Participants receive considerable instinctual information from the imageries and symbols without you having to interpret for them. Their inner wisdom or subconscious mind will take them where they need to go. The more you let go of any need to direct their experiences, or feel that you are responsible to interpret, the better.

You can always ask, even when using the Universal Symbol Dictionary, "Does that resonate with you?" This empowers participants to come to their own conclusions about the significance of the imagery, and it allows you to simply be the guide and a partner on their journey.

Over the years, I've learned that the best interpreter of imagery is *always* the participant who just experienced it. Simply asking questions and maintaining a conversation will elicit expression of the participant's own inner wisdom. It will empower them and encourage their respect for their innate intelligence.

HAVE FUN WITH IT!

Imagery is not only healing, insightful, and integrating, it can also be funny at times. People's imaginations are overflowing with humorous images. It's always a positive surprise to hear someone in a group who was previously solemn break into peals of laughter, or to watch as a participant's face bursts into a smile during an imagery. Laughter is healing and brings people together. Imagery is like other imagining, except one's eyes are usually closed. Laughter is allowed!

STEP-BY-STEP IMAGERY PROCESS

1. Prepare environment (safe, quiet, confidential, phones off).
2. Read Relaxation, Imagery and "Awakening" from Imagery Page.
3. Give participant(s) 5-10 seconds to readjust after opening their eyes from imagery.
4. Begin to read/ask numbered Insight Page Questions from adjacent Insight Page. You can have the participant verbally answer the questions one after the other as you ask them, or you can read questions aloud and have the participant or group members write all the answers down and discuss after they are finished.
5. After the participant answers questions, you can tell them the symbolic focus of the imagery, if it has one. (Example: Car=self, Sword=masculinity, Vase=femininity). Once they understand the connection, you can discuss their experience at a deeper level.

GET CREATIVE

1. Have participants write down their imagery experience and then share verbally. Many participants want a written memory of the imagery which they can revisit at a later date to possibly receive more information from.
2. Have participants draw or create a collage from their imagery or create an imagery journal.
3. Write your own imagery based on your goal or create a workshop around a particular imagery subject. Example: I do an imagery where participants visualize a symbol that represents "Joy in Sobriety." I give them an outline of a mandala, (circles within circles) and have them draw the symbol they visualized in the middle of the mandala, then other symbols of their choice outside the symbol. Their drawing and meanings are discussed after completion.
4. Have groups break into dyads to share their imagery experience.
5. Utilize the Adaptations for select imageries listed in the Purpose Boxes.
6. Record yourself reading the imagery of your choice; listen, then answer questions and journal about the experience.

DIFFERENT WAYS TO FACILITATE IMAGERY

IMAGERY FACILITATION	DESCRIPTION	EXAMPLE F = Facilitator, P = Participant
PASSIVE IMAGERY (individual or groups) Benefit: Participant relaxation.	• Participant is non-verbal, while listening to facilitator and imagining. • For individual or group work.	**F:** "You're in the most beautiful place, becoming very relaxed." **P:** Listens only.
PARTIALLY ACTIVE IMAGERY (individual or groups) Benefit: Facilitator knows when to move forward in imagery.	• Facilitator asks participant(s) for input when needed. • Can be done with one client or smaller group.	**F:** "When you're in your safe place, let me know by nodding your head or saying yes." **P:** Nods, and facilitator continues.
PASSIVE (SYMBOLIC) IMAGERY with PREPARED QUESTIONS Benefit: Participant receives personal attention, debriefing, and understanding of the imagery.	• Participant is non-verbal during imagery. • Facilitator asks questions regarding imagery, after imagery is complete, to assist in participants' understanding.	**F:** "Ask your guide for the answer. And say goodbye for now." **P:** Listens only. **AFTER IMAGERY:** **F:** Asks prepared questions of participant to assist in deeper understanding of imagery.
INTERACTIVE IMAGERY(SM) Benefit: Because the participant and facilitator have fluid verbal interaction during the imagery, the facilitator can follow the participants lead, to guide the participant where they need/want to go.	• Participant and facilitator have verbal interaction *during* imagery. • The participant directs, and the facilitator follows. (The next step depends on the participant's response.)	**F:** "And where are you now?" **P:** "I'm floating in a boat on a small bay." **F:** "What's happening there?" **P:** "It's very peaceful. There's a mermaid in the water who wants my attention." **F:** "What would you like to do?" **P:** "I'd like to get in the water and speak with her." **F:** "Okay, go ahead and do that now."

*Author's note: This book focuses on passive symbolic imagery.

WHAT TO DO IF . . .

Note: It is rare to have negative reactions to imagery. Imagery is a safe and gentle modality in which to release emotion. In my experience, I find the situations below to be the exceptions, not the norm.

THIS HAPPENS	ACTION TO TAKE
Crying / Emoting	**Crying:** Allow the participant to emote. Ask them what brought on the emotion. Most people are relieved to release their feelings and be heard and understood. The calming effect of imagery provides a soft and soothing approach to releasing grief and sadness. **Intense crying:** Ask the participant if they're okay and allow them to emote until they are able to express their feelings. If you are in a group situation where the participant has access to a personal counselor or therapist outside the group, and they choose to leave, allow them to connect with their personal therapist.
Participant says, "I don't see anything."	Ask, "If you did see something, what would you see?" The participant might process kinesthetically (through feelings and/or the body) or auditorily (through hearing) in the way they imagine; however, ninety-nine percent of the time, this question works and they have an answer to it. If it doesn't work, you could ask, "What do you feel you would see?" or "Do you sense anything?" or "Do you hear anything?" This usually opens up the imagination, and you can walk them through the imagery again; they'll follow and continue on.
Participant says, "I have no idea what the symbol means."	First ask, "What is the first thing you think of when I say [the symbol]?" Assure them that there is no wrong answer in the imagination. Give them some time to process and express their thoughts and feelings about the symbol. Then continue by asking, "And how does that relate to the subject of (imagery)?" See Chapter 4, Symbols, for more questions to ask to assist participant.
Participant begins laughing during individual or group imagery	Almost everyone has experienced suppressed laughter. You're in a group environment, and one simple thing sets you off and you're laughing and can't stop! Laughter is a healthy release of stress that sends endorphins coursing through the body. I was once doing a hypnosis demonstration for a class, when the hypnosis volunteer began to laugh uncontrollably. It was a perfect teaching moment. I told the volunteer, "Just let yourself laugh. It's a great stress relief!" After her laughter calmed (and it took a while!), she let out a long, loud sigh, and said, "I've been so stressed lately—and that felt so good!"

THIS HAPPENS	ACTION TO TAKE
Participant opens eyes	**Individual:** The participant might be anxious, feel like they can't concentrate, or possibly feel intimidated. I tell them it is fine to leave their eyes open. They usually feel better about having a choice, and then they close their eyes again and resume following the imagery. Some participants who have experienced trauma might want to keep their eyes open during imagery. This is rare, but it does happen. I tell them that it is absolutely fine to keep their eyes open during imagery. They can imagine with their eyes open; they do it every day. **Group:** As you need to continue reading/facilitating the imagery with the group, allow the person to leave their eyes open (if you can, gesture that it's okay). If needed, talk with them after the imagery is complete. The issue might be anxiety or previous trauma, so follow the recommendations above. Just giving a person the choice to leave their eyes open normally relaxes them.
Participant seems resistant to imagery	I first allow the participant to express their feelings and opinions about imagery. Oftentimes, people have resistance because they don't know what imagery entails and feel uncomfortable with the unknown. They might say, "I can't do this" or "I can't see anything!" I never push; I gently guide them by using some of the methods above, such as, "If you did see something, what would you see?" or ask them what they find difficult about it. One of the most resistant participants I ever encountered became one of my most enthusiastic students because I allowed her to express her opposition. She was in a class I was teaching, which was required by her employer. When I asked her what she wanted to learn, she explained, "Nothing. I'm here because I have to be." I asked her to be the first volunteer for imagery. Immediately after the imagery, she opened her eyes, and with a big smile on her face, said, "I loved that!" Generally, after allowing a person to express their feelings, they are more open to trying imagery. If not, honor that. Not every person likes or wants to experience imagery, and that is fine. I have found, however, that most people find it extremely relaxing, interesting, or insightful after they have experienced it.

CHAPTER 4
SYMBOLS

DEFINITION

Simply put, a symbol is a thing that represents or stands for something else. Symbols can have simple or complex meanings. They can be abstract. And they can have multiple levels of meaning.

"The language and the 'people' of the unconscious are symbols, and the means of communication, dreams." [9] The beauty is that we don't have to go to sleep in order to dream, to connect with our deeper mind. We can access symbols in the waking state through imagery, which can be easily remembered and then interpreted.

SYMBOLS: THE LANGUAGE OF THE SUBCONSCIOUS

Our subconscious mind creates symbols from our feelings and beliefs. Symbols and imagination are the *language* of the subconscious. And because symbols bypass the conscious mind, they also bypass judgment and denial, making them a wonderful therapeutic tool. They can bring up unconscious material that can assist the participant and practitioner to move forward in understanding and move toward needed change.

Many people visualize mystical, mythical beings, as well as people known and unknown that come to bring information.

Anything can be a symbol brimming with information: nature, shapes, sounds, colors, numbers, etc. I think of imagery as seeing with our "inside eyes" or with the "eyes of the soul" that feel and sense as well as see. Through imagery, we create waking dreams to visualize symbols for specific purposes.

INTERPRETING SYMBOLS

In the pages ahead, you'll learn how to ask simple questions to help participants further interpret imagery symbols. Participants might not realize it initially, but they often already know what the symbols they visualize mean. Asking the right questions and keeping the conversation going will bring the meaning to their conscious awareness.

TWO TYPES OF SYMBOLS: PERSONAL AND UNIVERSAL

Always, the first and most important symbol to interpret is the personal symbol. Symbols are *very* personal for each individual and can also have different meanings within cultures. Therefore, it is of primary importance to allow the participant to fully share their perception of the symbol first.

9   Carl C. Jung, Man and His Symbols, (Bantam Doubleday, 1964), pp. Introduction, viii, John Freeman

PERSONAL SYMBOLS

A personal symbol is a symbol that has a very specific meaning to an individual based on that person's past experiences and beliefs.

Example: Dog = Unconditional love   *or*

Dog = Fear

A dog can mean unconditional love and loyalty to one person; to another, who was bitten as a child, it can signify fear. The meaning is personal to the individual. This is the most important information for the participant to receive.

PERSONAL INTERPRETATION

First, ask the questions aloud from the Insight page and have the participant answer verbally. The participant will receive much more information by expressing their experience **in their own language**. Depending on your process, you can also have the participant(s) write down their answers and then read them aloud. Their answers will generate important information based on their personal interpretation. When in groups, I ask each individual to share their answers with the group and I take notes so I have the information they're sharing.

UNIVERSAL SYMBOLS

A Universal symbol means the same thing to most cultures, ages, and people worldwide.

Example: Peace Sign = Peace

Butterfly = Transformation

Heart = Love

In the most basic sense, these symbols are defined by the universal meanings above.

UNIVERSAL INTERPRETATION

Example: Heart = Love

"What else does it mean to you?"

Amir sees a huge heart that shines with ambient light. He says it means love. When asked, "What else does it mean to you?" He says, "I give my heart out easily, and I feel really vulnerable now."

In this case, it involves his love and emotions and holds true to the universal meaning. You can still continue to ask further questions regarding the *personal meaning* from the participant, as asked of Amir.

WORD ASSOCIATION: CONNECTING THE DOTS

Utilize word association to elicit further information from the participant:

Example: Giraffe = Tall, can see far into the distance.

"How does that relate to your life?"

The participant says, "I have no idea why I saw a giraffe; it means nothing to me." You can ask, "When I say the word *giraffe*, what is the first thing you think of?" This will start the conversation that unfolds into greater understanding. The participant might associate *giraffe* with the word *tall*, or the idea that *giraffes can see far into the distance*. Continue asking questions, such as, "How does seeing into the distance relate to your present life?"

The more you connect the dots through the questions you ask, and the answers they give, the more you can assist the participant in discovering deeper meaning.

Remember that it's much more important that they resonate with their personal meaning than what you might interpret it as.

It's not your job to interpret for them. Your questions will lead them to their own insights. If they don't resonate with *anything* that comes up in conversation, go to the Universal Symbol Dictionary (USD) in the back of the book to see if they resonate with that description, or if it moves them forward in understanding.

Example: Stop Sign = Stop using drugs

Mary says, "I saw a stop sign on the front of my t-shirt."

Even though this symbol generally means *stop* to most people (universally), we are always interested in getting the personal interpretation. When asked, "What does this mean to you personally?" or "How does this relate to your present life right now?" Mary replies, "It means stop using drugs."
Again, if the participant cannot relate to the symbol at all after using word association (this is rare), look up the universal meaning in the USD. Let them know that the definition *tends* to mean this. Ask them if the qualities related to their symbol have meaning for them or relate to them in any way. Don't feel that you, or they, must know the interpretation immediately. Oftentimes, the meaning will unfold for them organically over time. Imagery often evokes layers of information and meanings. I have had clients leave my office with no idea of what a particular imagery meant to them and then return a week later with amazing connections and insights.

If you are working with a group and have time, after *fully* discussing the meaning of an imagery with an individual, you can invite others in the group to share any insights about how the symbol might relate to their peer. This can be especially beneficial in a group that is well-acquainted and well-bonded. The feedback is normally appreciated by the individual, and they are free to resonate with only what feels right to them.

Again, **do not feel that you must know the interpretation**. The meaning will often unfold for the participant in their own time.

Though people generally *know* the essence and meaning of the symbols they see, they might not realize it initially. The questions they answer on the Insight page will elicit basic information. Then they can discover deeper meaning(s) by answering the questions *you* ask.

Trust the subconscious. It is brilliant!

INTERPRETING DISTINCT QUALITIES OF SYMBOLS

QUESTIONS TO ASK

The subconscious speaks through symbols and gives us messages through the symbols' qualities. **We discover the meaning of a symbol by expressing words that describe it.** Listen to the words that the participant uses to describe their images.

SIZE

The larger the symbol, the more it wants your attention.

A large symbol has significant information for you. Sometimes, after a participant has dialogued with a large symbol and given it the attention it wanted, it will shrink in size. The size can also denote the power you give to what the symbol represents, or the power it has in your life.

Example: (Large)   Very large bell = Attention called to education

Malia sees a huge bell that's ringing in a school tower. When asked, "What does the bell mean to you?" Malia answers, "I'm not sure, but it's really, really big!" When asked, "What does the school tower mean to you?" she replies, "I really want to finish my degree." Then she mentions that, "Maybe the school bell is calling me back to college." After she talks more about her desire to finish school, she says that she is now seeing the bell in her imagination as normal sized.

A small symbol does not mean that the message is insignificant. If an object is smaller than its life-size form, this can mean that it's unimportant to you, or that you're not giving it value.

Example: (Small)   Tiny Wedding Ring = Unsure of Marriage

Justin visualized his wife's wedding ring, but it was tiny compared to its real-life size. Though it was very small, it was glowing and sparkling with light that caught Justin's attention. His eyes began to tear up as he said, "I'm not sure whether my wife wants to stay married. I haven't been there for her in a long time."

SHAPE

First, ask the participant, "What does this shape mean to you?" and "How does it make you feel?" (The personal meaning). Continue following that line of questioning with them.

If they're having a hard time understanding it, ask, "What are the first words that come to your mind when you see this shape?"

After you feel that they understand its personal meaning, you can choose to look up the shape in the Universal Symbol Dictionary (USD) in the back of the book. Some of the shapes listed include square, rectangle, arrow, circle, oval, line, triangle, diamond, star, etc. The meanings given relate to the qualities the symbol possesses.

Example: Arrow = Up

Up = Optimism

"How does this relate to your life?"
"How I like to be."

Antoinette sees an arrow pointing upward. When asked what it means to her, she replies, "It means *up*." She is then asked, "What does the word *up* mean to you?"

She replies, "An up person. Someone optimistic."

When asked, "How does this relate to you in your life?" Antoinette says, "That's what I like to be, and I think that's how people see me."

Example: Sphere with spikes

"How does it make you feel?
"Anxious."

Alma sees a round sphere with spikes in it in her stomach. She says she's not sure what it means. When asked, "How does the shape make you feel?" she says, "Kind of anxious. I think it's about me worrying too much and how it makes my stomach hurt." She nods and says, "Yeah, the spikes are all the things I worry about. If I stopped worrying, there would just be a smooth circle in my stomach."

COLOR

Colors have distinct meanings to individuals.

First ask, "What does the color represent to you?" and "How does the color make you feel?"

Then ask, "What are the first words that come to your mind when you think of the color (blue)?"

If more information is desired, look in the USD (Universal Symbol Dictionary).

Note: Black and white (together) are commonly seen in imagery. First ask, "What do those colors mean to you?" Ask what meaning resonates with the participant. If they are unaware, check the USD.

(In the universal sense, black and white together can denote all-or-nothing thinking, or duality, as in day and night, yin and yang, etc.)

Example: Red musical note in heart = Passion / Career

Reginald sees a brilliant red musical note in his heart. He says it represents his love of music, and the color red reminds him of passion. The musical note begins to move around as if it's dancing and reminds him of how music brings him happiness. He says his love of music is his passion and that he's thinking of making it his career.

TEXTURE

Ask the participant about the texture. Is the texture of the symbol soft, smooth, hard, uneven, rough, or spiked?

These textures range from ease toward difficulty, from comfort toward discomfort. The texture of the symbol relates to the ease or difficulty of the subject of the imagery.

Example: Spikey Cross = Spirituality / Judgmental

"What is judgmental about spirituality?"
"Relative judged me."

Alisha saw a cross that was metallic and spikey. She said the cross represented her spirituality. She commented that she didn't want to get too close to it because of the spikes. She felt it was judgmental but wasn't sure why.

The practitioner connected the dots by asking Alisha, "What is judgmental about spirituality?" After some discussion, she said that she has been avoiding a relative who had judged her for being of a different faith.

CLARITY

How clear or unclear the symbol is can determine how close (physically or emotionally), understood, or intimate what it represents is to the person visualizing it.

CLEAR: When a symbol is very clear and easy to see, it usually indicates that the participant easily connects with the subject it represents or sees it clearly.

Example: Mother = Clear

Lily sees her mother, to whom she was very close. Though her mother has been gone for years, she sees her mother as "crystal clear" and can feel her strong presence.

UNCLEAR: If the symbol is opaque or almost invisible, it *can* mean that what it represents is unclear at present, hard to understand, or invisible in the person's life. (An exception to this could be if a "spirit" is seen as transparent, and this feels appropriate for the person visualizing it.)

Example: In circle with children = Unclear

"What is unclear about this circle?"
"Unsure of how I want to work with children."

Kayla sees herself in the middle of a circle with young children. She says she isn't sure what she's doing there, and the scene is unclear. When asked, "What is unclear about this circle of children?" Kayla replies, "I'd like to work with kids someday, but I'm not sure in what way yet." This thought generates an idea for Kayla, and she says, "I think I'm going to check into that!"

CARTOON

Occasionally a person will see an image in cartoon-form, such as an animal, person, or actual cartoon character. This can mean several things:

- They are making "light" of a situation/person to better deal with it.
- They aren't taking the issue seriously or handling it in a mature way.
- They are afraid of the situation or person.
- They identify with the aspects/qualities of the actual cartoon character.

Example 1: Tony the Tiger = Strong = "Stronger than you think"

Bill saw Tony the Tiger, who was strong and assertive. He said that Tony the Tiger gave him the message, "You're stronger than you think! Get up and gooo!"

Bill laughs, because he says his older brother, who was very supportive of him, used to talk like Tony the Tiger in a cartoon voice. It reminds him that he can get through things that he sometimes thinks he can't.

Example 2: Cartoon prince = Fantasy

Jenny visualized her ex-boyfriend as a cartoon prince who rides in on a horse to rescue her. When asked, "In what way do you think of your ex-boyfriend as a cartoon prince?" Jenny replies, "Well, I thought he was perfect when I met him. He was always helping me, and I thought he loved me, but then he started getting angry and abusive. He wasn't who I thought he was."

In this case, Jenny had idealized her boyfriend, and he was more of a fantasy (cartoon) than real. It can also be easier to visualize and deal with a cartoon character of a person whom one fears or has been hurt by.

PLACEMENT

Where or how an image is placed can give you important information.

Example 1: Cube on corner = Vulnerable

Darius sees a large cube that represents his life at present. He says it is balanced precariously on one corner instead of resting flat on the ground. The practitioner asks, "How do you feel about that?" Darius says, "Well, it feels unbalanced. It's on edge. It could fall over."

The practitioner then asks, "And how does that relate to you?"

Darius replies, "I think I feel kind of vulnerable, like the cube. I'm starting a new job in a new city, and I don't feel settled yet."

Note: Tipping, leaning, and changing of balance all indicate a motion toward change. The feeling that the participant has about the motion indicates their feeling about the change. Though many people would interpret this as unbalanced or vulnerable, it could also be interpreted as unique or risky by another person who feels positively about it. This is the importance of always getting the personal interpretation first and honoring it.

Example 2: Father as horse in distance = Distant even when present

Violet sees her father as a horse standing off in the distance in a pasture. The practitioner asks, "How do you feel about the horse standing in the distance?" Violet replies, "My dad's never around, and when he is, he's still distant. It's disappointing." The practitioner then asks, "And how does that relate to you in your present life?" Violet says, "I have to stop pretending he's going to change and accept him for who he is."

MOTION

A symbol might be in motion—moving forward, turning, spinning, pulsating, and changing patterns, color, or size.

When a symbol moves, there is added meaning in its motion. You can ask the participant several questions about it. Is it moving up and down? Forward and back? In which direction, from left to right or right to left? It can mean that what the symbol represents is alive, that it wants your attention, or that its message to you is within the movement itself.

Example 1:
Rabbit hopping forward, backward = Slow movement forward

Erik sees a rabbit that represents his goal to open his own business. He's confused about why he saw a rabbit. When explaining the rabbit to the practitioner, he describes how he watched the rabbit hop forward, then turn around and hop backwards, turn around again, and then hop farther forward.

He says, "It was eventually getting somewhere, but not very fast."

The practitioner asks him, "How does that relate to your goal of opening your business?"

Erik replies, "Well, it seems like every time I make some progress, something pulls me back and distracts me. But I do keep moving forward. I guess maybe it's a message that I just need to keep working toward it whenever I can."

Example 2:
Turning heart changing colors = Confusion and vulnerability

In an imagery focused on love, Ali visualizes a glass heart that is slowly turning. It is also continuously changing from red to blue and blue to red.

When asked, "How does the turning glass heart make you feel?" he replies, "It's confusing, I'm not sure what it means."

The practitioner connects the dots by asking, "What is confusing about love?"

Ali says, "Well, I never know how my girlfriend feels. She keeps changing her mind about our relationship. I think that's why the heart is changing colors from red to blue. I always say that she runs hot and cold." After more discussion, Ali says, "The heart is glass because that's how I feel with her. Breakable."

This brings up more discussion about where Ali wants to go with his relationship.

SOUND

Ask the participant how the sound makes them feel. The sound could be soft, loud, beautiful, humming, haunting, annoying, or even frightening. The relevance is what feeling the sound generates and if it is related to a specific memory.

Example 1: Dove cooing = Calming

Brook hears the sound of a dove cooing in her imagery. She says it makes her think of her childhood and summers by the lake. She says it calms and relaxes her and she loves it.

Example 2: Ice clinking = Hypervigilance to wife's drinking

Kyle hears the sound of ice clinking in a glass and says it makes his body tense up. When the practitioner asks, "Do you know how that sound relates to your body tensing up?" he says, "It reminds me of when I was hypervigilant about my wife's drinking." The practitioner continues questioning by asking, "And how does this relate to you presently?" Kyle answers, "It reminds me that I have to let go of her behavior and focus on my own life."

SCENT

Scent is our most primitive sense. It can bring back memories instantaneously.

Ask the participant, "How does this scent make you feel?" You can also ask, "What words or thoughts come to mind with this scent?"

Smell can reconnect us to our memories more quickly than any other sense. Certain scents can influence our mood in a positive or negative way.

Example: Night-blooming jasmine = Family time together
= Simple things

Azita smells night-blooming jasmine in her imagery, which she says was her mother's favorite scent.

When asked how it makes her feel, she says, "It's comforting and bittersweet at the same time because I miss my mom. It also brings back happy times of my family in the house I grew up in." When asked, "If the scent had a message for you, what would it be?" Azita says, "To find joy in the simple things, like family and time together."

SYMBOLS CAN BE VISUAL LANGUAGE

Example: Large face = Facing a situation
Impatiens flower = Impatient

- Picturing a large face can literally mean *facing a situation* and would refer to the subject of the imagery.
- Seeing an impatiens flower in an imagery could refer (literally) to being impatient and needing patience regarding the subject of the imagery. Another example could be seeing a *porpoise* that tells you

your *purpose* (i.e. words that are known as *near homophones* because they are close in sound but not in spelling or meaning).
- Visualizing a ham might be a message about *hamming it up*.

The participant can receive the message as they speak the words describing the symbol. The more they verbalize their experience, the better the chances of them understanding its meaning.

VISUAL, AUDITORY, AND KINESTHETIC INTAKE

VISUAL

We all take in sensory information differently through our five senses. Though we use all of our senses, we have preferred ways in which we take in the outside world. Have you ever heard a person say, "I see what you're saying"? It's not that they actually *saw* what you were saying, but that person's preferred representational system (or the way they take in information) is most likely visual.

Visual people tend to use visual language: words such as *see, imagine, look, picture, notice*. Because their primary intake is visual, they use visual words to communicate what they experience and understand. These people also experience imagery primarily through *seeing* it in their imaginations.

Example: "*Saw* a dolphin swimming"

"*Looked* at me"

"*Image* of swimming together."

Anha describes her imagery by saying, "I **saw** a dolphin that was swimming through the water toward me. It swam right to me and **looked** up at me. I could **see** it was happy, and I got an **image** of the dolphin and me swimming together."

KINESTHETIC

Others, who are more kinesthetic (they feel and understand through their bodies), take in their information through sensing and feeling. They might just *sense* and *feel* what an imagery means, without as much, or any, visualization at all. These people use language such as *I feel, in touch with, hold, grasp*, etc. Also, the information they receive in imagery might not be complete *while* experiencing it. They might continue to sense it and let it percolate until the meaning becomes clear to them.

Example: "*Feeling* presence"

"I *sensed*"

"*Feels* right"

Emilio **feels a presence** that represents a spiritual guide in imagery. He explains that, "I couldn't see its face, but I **sensed** that it knew me well." After some time, Emilio says that, "It felt like a combination of God and my dad, who passed away five years ago." When asked why he imagined them together, he replied, "Well, it just **feels right** that my dad would be with God, and my dad always hoped that I would believe in God too."

<u>AUDITORY</u>

Auditory people prefer gaining their information through hearing words. They also relate to internal dialogue while processing information. They use language such as *tell me, explain it, sounds good to me,* and *I hear you.* Within imagery, they often *hear* messages through their imagination.

Example: "*Heard* beautiful music"

"*Explained*"

"*Sounded* good"

Michael describes his imagery experience: "I **heard** this beautiful music coming from the top of the hill. I walked to the top and **heard** a voice that **explained** that because music is my passion, I should find a way to make it my career. That **sounded good** to me."

ADDITIONAL QUESTIONS TO ASK FOR INTERPRETATION

ADDITIONAL QUESTIONS TO ASK (to add to Insight Page Questions)

To be used if the participant is having trouble answering the questions, or to simply get more information.

1. "What does the [symbol] mean to you?"
2. "What is the first thing that comes to your mind when you hear the word [insert word here]?"
3. "Anything else?"
4. "How does this relate to your present life?"
5. "And how does that relate to [subject of imagery, relationship, goals, or the subject the participant brought up]?"
6. "If the symbol had a message for you, what would it be?"
7. After all questions asked: "What action can you take from the information you received?"

Example: Diamond's many facets

Q: **"What does a diamond mean to you?"**
A: "I'm not sure . . ."

Q: **"What is the first thing that comes to your mind when you hear the word diamond?"**
A: "Special."

Q: **"Anything else?"**
A: "Well, I think each diamond is unique. They're sparkly, beautiful, and they have many facets to them."

Q: **"How does this relate to your present life?"**
A: "I'm working on improving my self-esteem. And I do have many facets to my personality."

Q: **"How does that relate to relationships (the subject of imagery)?"**
A: "I want to feel special in my relationship and be treated with respect."

Q: **"If the diamond had a message for you, what would it be?"**
A: "Treat me like a diamond, like I'm precious and special.

Q: **"Is there a positive action you can take at this time?"**
A: "Well, I could talk to my fiance about my feelings."

Example: Possums play dead

Ask the participant these questions if they answer, "I don't know." In this example, the participant has said that he saw a possum as the symbol of Health and Sobriety.

Q: **"What does a possum mean to you?"**
A: "I don't have any idea. Nothing, really."

Q: **"What is the first thing that comes to your mind? Just say it out loud."**
A: "I think they play dead, right? When they're in danger?"

Q: **"And how does that relate to you and sobriety?"**
A: "Umm . . . when I'm using, I isolate. I don't return phone calls, I don't see my family. I guess I kind of play dead. That's probably why the possum said, 'You can stop now.'"

HOW TO USE THE UNIVERSAL SYMBOL DICTIONARY (USD)

1. **THE USD IS AN ALPHABETICAL LIST OF OVER 500 SYMBOLS** which might be encountered within the imageries. The meanings are the symbol's *attributes* and *qualities* as universal interpretations and are not meant to be predictive.

2. I also created a **QUICK REFERENCE USD OF COMMON SYMBOLS**. This is located at the back of the book, directly behind the USD. It will assist you to quickly find the following imagery themes:

   - Animals
   - Birds
   - Body
   - Chakras
   - Colors
   - Directions
   - Elements
   - Fish/Sea Life
   - Flowers
   - Food
   - House/Rooms
   - Insects
   - Landscapes
   - Metals
   - Numbers
   - Shapes
   - Stones/Gems
   - Trees
   - Waterscapes
   - Weather

3. As I've said before and repeat often: <u>always have the participant verbalize their personal interpretation of their imagery first</u>. Use the Insight Page, ask additional questions, and then expand upon it by referring to the USD.

4. If the participant has no idea of what the symbol means, even after you've asked additional questions, look up the symbol in the USD to see if it resonates with them.

5. People have asked me if they can use the USD to interpret dreams. The answer is yes, of course you can! Symbols are symbols whether they come from dreams (sleeping), visions (awake), or from imagery (relaxed while awake). They all arise from the subconscious mind.

6. If you don't find a symbol in the USD, you can check the internet by typing the words *symbology* or *symbolism* after the name of the symbol. You will get many definitions—choose the one that you most resonate with or the participant finds most meaningful.

CHAPTER 5
THE 52 GUIDED IMAGERIES

IMAGERY	PURPOSE	DESCRIPTION	PAGE
Ancestor	Relationships, Family Values	Connect and dialogue with an ancestor	52
Animal Adventure	Self-Discovery	Have an adventure as an animal.	54
Animal as Health and Sobriety	Addiction, Sobriety	Beliefs about health and/or sobriety through discussion with animal	56
Animal Representing	Clarity	Dialogue with an animal about an emotion, issue or quality	58
Animals as Parents	Relationships, Family	Meet two animals representing parents, and receive a message	60
Animals Head and Stomach	Self-Awareness	Reveal thoughts and emotions and their interplay	62
Backpack	Release, Self-Care	Choose whether to release a burden	64
Bird	Confidence	Experience a goal as accomplished	66
Bridge Across the River	Grief, Inspiration	Dialogue with a separated loved one	68
Canyon	Motivation	Overcome obstacle to attain a goal	70
Car	Self-Awareness	Discover values, desires, needs	72
Cavern	Addiction, Sobriety	Visualize and dialogue with addiction	74
Child Expected	Relationships, Child	Connect with the child you expect	76
Childhood Home	Childhood Issues	Visit your childhood home	78

IMAGERY	PURPOSE	DESCRIPTION	PAGE
Circle of Support	Confidence	Verbal support through celebration	80
Coat	Release	Choose to keep or release protection	82
Creative Self	Creativity	Connect to Creativity	84
Crying Child	Inner Child	Re-parent Inner Child	86
Cube	Self-Discovery	Connect with self, support system, love, challenges	88
Director	Relationships	Honest communication in relationship	90
Forest of Forgiveness	Forgiveness	Forgive another or yourself	92
Future Self	Motivation	Experience yourself as you wish to be	94
Garden of Gratitude	Acceptance, Gratitude	Express gratitude to another	96
Guide	Self-Discovery	Meet a wise, supportive guide	98
Hall of False Beliefs	Release, Self-love	Reframe and rename a false belief	100
Healing Temple	Health, Wellness	Visit a healing temple	102
Healthy Self	Health, Wellness	Embody Health, Energy, Wellness	104
Higher Power / Higher Self	Faith, Spirituality	Connect with Higher Power / Higher Self	106
Horse	Relationships, Trust	Trust and openness in relationships	108
House	Self-Discovery	Examine aspects of yourself	110
Judge	Clarity, Self-Love	Visualize yourself as your judge	112
Library	Self-Awareness	Connect with your values, goals and interests	114
Life's Dream Inn	Inspiration	Live your life's dream	116

IMAGERY	PURPOSE	DESCRIPTION	PAGE
Masquerade	Self-Awareness	Become aware of the mask you wear	118
Mountain	Self-Awareness, Motivation	Rise above your challenges	120
Power Source	Confidence	Embody your own power	122
Purpose	Inspiration, Motivation	Embody your purpose	124
Rain	Being Present	Renewal through cleansing	126
Return to the Future	Inner Child	Healing inner child	128
River	Being Present	Anchor in relaxation response	130
Room Representing	Self-Discovery	Rearrange a room representing challenge	132
Stars	Abundance, Creativity	Mentally create your desire	134
Swimming with Sealife	Being Present	Be present, connect with sea life	136
Sword and Vase	Relationships	Masculinity / Femininity	138
Symbol of Your Life	Self-Awareness	Perception of life at present.	140
T-Shirt	Clarity	What you present and what you feel	142
Talk With the Body	Release	Dialogue with an issue through your body	144
Transformation	Inspiration, Motivation	Attend a Ceremony of Transition	146
Tree	Being Present	Experience yourself as a tree	148
Two Roads	Awareness, Release	Visit past and future with guide	150
Welcome	Self-Love	Connect with your newborn self	152
Wellspring	Creativity	Connect to Creativity	154

IMAGERIES BY PURPOSE

Though each imagery has a primary purpose shown on pages 41-43, all of the imageries contain many different purposes as listed below:

ACCEPTANCE / ALLOWANCE / TRUST

ADDICTION / SOBRIETY

BEING PRESENT

CHILDHOOD / INNER CHILD

CLARITY

CONFIDENCE

FAITH / SPIRITUALITY

FORGIVENESS

GRIEF

HEALTH

INSPIRATION / MOTIVATION

RELEASE

HOW TO USE THE IMAGERY PAGE

ANIMAL REPRESENTING . . .

"Animals are such agreeable friends—they ask no questions, they pass no criticisms." ~ George Eliot

With this imagery, choose an emotion, issue, or quality you want to address, such as love, joy, compassion, sadness, fear, anger, addiction, transition, decision, acceptance, courage, loyalty, etc.

Relaxing into the surface you're on . . . Allowing your body to relax into gravity . . . Closing your eyes as you're ready . . . Taking in a deep, healing breath as you allow all your muscles to expand and let go, slowing down by taking another healing breath and releasing that. Gently breathing into your stomach and up into your chest . . . and exhaling . . . with complete permission to relax and rest . . . into the stillness of the moment, into your center, in the here and now. Breathing in and out . . . and out and in . . . as breathing becomes slower and deeper . . . and rhythmic . . . And you shift your attention inward into the imagination . . . Where you find yourself standing in front of a small lake . . . that glitters under the sun . . . You smell the fresh, clean smell of earth and hear the trees gently rustling in the breeze . . .

BRIEF INDUCTION / RELAXATION:
Read slowly, pause at ellipses . . .

And now you see an animal that represents (emotion, issue, or quality).

(Note: Please pause after each question to allow the participant time to visualize and process.)

1. What animal is it? Look at its size and its color.
2. Notice its qualities.
3. What is your impression of this animal?
4. What condition is it in?
5. What does this animal think of you?
6. What do you like about it? And dislike?
7. And now, become the animal.
8. What do you experience as the animal?
9. And as the animal, what do you think of you, the person?
10. And now, become yourself again.
11. The animal has a message for you. Just listen: you might hear it or intuitively know what the message is.

Thank the animal in whatever way you choose for the information it brought.

IMAGERY:
Make sure to pause after each question. Read slowly, calmly, with inflection.

And now, beginning to focus your attention on the outside world again, as you hear the sounds around you . . . Feeling the surface under you . . . Feeling comfortable and content, focused and refreshed. Remembering everything you saw and experienced . . . Beginning to stretch your fingers and toes, counting up one and two . . . Feeling peaceful and content as you return to awareness . . . More aware and alert, three . . . and four . . . And on the count of five, opening your eyes to the light of the room, refreshed, relaxed, and aware . . .

BRIEF AWAKENING:
Begin reading a bit louder, pick up pace and energy. Give the participant time to adjust after opening their eyes before asking questions from the Insight Page.

REMINDERS:

- Assure confidentiality.
- Maintain a calm, quiet space.
- Turn off all phones.
- Make sure the participant is ready.
- Use your voice as a tool.

HOW TO USE THE INSIGHT PAGE

DIALOGUE WITH ANIMAL ABOUT EMOTION, ISSUE, OR QUALITY

PURPOSE: *SELF-DISCOVERY*

SUMMARY: Participant visualizes an animal. They have a dialogue, receive a message, and become the animal, to experience greater understanding.

MY EXPERIENCE: Even those who aren't animal lovers feel safe as they connect to animals within imagery. I often witness people visualizing animals that they are very unfamiliar with, and are surprised to see, but there's always an important factor in why this particular animal shows up to give the person a message.

EXAMPLE: Ashly sees a large, silly bear that represents fear, which she finds surprising and a bit comical. Becoming the bear gives Ashly a feeling of strength and a feeling of levity at the irony. She receives the message, "It's okay! Even bears get scared! You're stronger than you know." Ashly later says this reminds her that she's strong and inspires her to move through fear.

ADAPTATION: Any emotion, issue, or quality can be used with this animal imagery for self-discovery: fear, joy, resentment, gratitude, acceptance, health, codependency, love, independence, hope, etc.

PURPOSE BOX:

PURPOSE: Explains purpose of imagery.

SUMMARY: Summarizes the imagery.

MY EXPERIENCE: The author's overall observations on how this imagery is received by participants, and other helpful information.

EXAMPLE: One person's experience of this imagery.

ADAPTATION: Suggestions to adapt the imagery to other purposes.

ANIMAL REPRESENTING: INSIGHT PAGE QUESTIONS

1. What animal came to you to represent your (emotion, quality, person, or challenge)?
2. Describe its qualities: appearance . . . size . . . color . . . condition . . . attitude.
3. What did you sense about this animal?
4. How did it feel being near it? What did you like about it?
5. Was there anything you disliked about it?
6. What did it think of you?
7. If you became the animal, how did it feel?
8. As the animal, what did you think of you, the person?
9. What was its message regarding your issue or situation?
10. And what does this mean to you?
11. How can you best use this information in your present life?

INSIGHT PAGE QUESTIONS:

Numbered questions to ask of participant about their imagery experience.

ANCESTOR

"It was the kind of moon that I would want to send back to my ancestors and gift to my descendants so they know that I too, have been bruised . . . by beauty." ~ Sanober Khan

Get settled into the surface you're on, close your eyes, and take in a long, deep healing breath. Inhale from your stomach up into your chest, and release the breath as you let go of all of the day's thoughts and concerns . . . Drifting down now into a soothing state of serenity . . . as your breathing slows . . . easily and naturally . . . exhaling anything unlike peace and calm. Feeling centered, calm, and content . . . as you rest into the stillness . . . within . . . into relaxation . . . with all senses soothed . . . drifting deeper . . . into the imagination, where you become aware that . . .

There is an important connection between you and an ancestor who shares your DNA. You might have been told about this person, know little about them, or simply imagine them, yet they are a part of you. Going deeper into your imaginal world, through the veil of time, you gently move back to meet this ancestor, in their land, in their time:

(Note: Please pause after each question to allow the participant time to visualize and process.)

1. Where do you find yourself? Look around. What do see here . . . and sense? (give ample time)
2. There in front of you appears your ancestor. How are they dressed?
3. Notice their build . . . their face . . . and their eyes. What do you see in their eyes?
4. Greet your ancestor in whatever way feels appropriate.
5. What is your first impression of them?
6. Ask your ancestor, "What kind of life have you lived?" (give ample time)
7. What were your goals and dreams? . . . Ask them if they realized their goals.
8. What qualities do you feel this relative has?
9. What qualities do you share?
10. What life lesson do you share?
11. Ask them what qualities and values they would like you to carry forward for posterity.
12. Ask them what they feel you should release for posterity.
13. Tell your ancestor what they have done that you are grateful for.
14. Your ancestor now tells you what they admire about you.
15. Thank your ancestor in whatever way you choose, and say good-bye, knowing you can always connect with them at another time.

And now beginning to return to the here and now . . . bringing back the information you received . . . with greater understanding . . . thankful to your ancestors for their strengths and sacrifice. Grateful for their mistakes and the lessons they received and passed on . . . Honoring the past and thankful for the present and all its possibilities . . . becoming more and more aware . . . as I count up 1 and 2 . . . feeling the surface under you . . . feeling grounded in the here and now . . . counting 3 . . . moving fingers and toes . . . stretching . . . counting 4 . . . and opening your eyes on the count of 5, relaxed and renewed, ready for the rest of the day.

MEET AN ANCESTOR

PURPOSE: *RELATIONSHIPS, FAMILY VALUES*

SUMMARY: Meet an ancestor in their time and environment. Discuss values and life purpose.

MY EXPERIENCE: People enjoy connecting with an ancestor they have heard about, know, or imagine. Most often, the participant projects their own values onto the ancestor and feels a bond with that person. If the ancestor has a questionable reputation, the participant has an opportunity to interpret their life from another perspective.

EXAMPLE: Brian connects with a Scottish man who is wearing a kilt. The man has long hair, a stocky build and a kind demeanor. He tells Brian that he raised sheep, farmed potatoes and lived a simple life. He said that he did the best with what he had, and found happiness. He told Brian to be honest, kind, and to appreciate those around him. The ancestor emphasized that he wished he had been educated and admired Brian for working hard. Brian is reminded of the gift of education and how it has impacted his life positively.

ANCESTOR: INSIGHT PAGE QUESTIONS:

1. Where were you?
2. What was the environment like? What did you sense there?
3. Describe the ancestor you saw: their build, their face, their eyes.
4. What did they wear? ... What did you see in their eyes?
5. How did you greet them?
6. What was your first impression of them?
7. What did they say about the life they lived?
8. Did they reach their desires?
9. What qualities did you notice in your ancestor?
10. What qualities do you share?
11. What life lesson do you share?
12. What qualities did they suggest you carry forward for posterity?
13. What did they suggest you release for posterity?
14. What did you thank them for?
15. What did they say they admire about you?
16. Did you receive a specific insight from experiencing this imagery?

ANIMAL ADVENTURE

"An animal's eyes have the power to speak a great language." ~ Martin Buber

Settling into the surface you're on . . . letting your body completely relax into gravity. Closing your eyes as you take in a deep, healing breath . . . into your stomach and up into your chest . . . Allowing all of your muscles to expand and let go . . . Slowing down, taking another breath, and releasing it. Gently breathing into your stomach and up into your chest and exhaling. Giving yourself complete permission to relax and rest into the stillness of the moment . . . Into your center, in the here and now. Gently breathing as your breath becomes slower . . . Shifting your attention inward, into the center of calm and contentment. Your mind and body at peace, as you move deeper into that center to allow yourself to wonder and wander . . . To drift down to observe and absorb the quiet . . . In the center . . . of the soothing . . . silence . . . within . . . Into the imagination . . . to the most open, natural space. Look around at the beauty. See the colors around you. Breathe in the fresh scents of nature. Feel the ground beneath your feet. Enjoy this moment of complete peace and quiet.

And now, invite a special animal to join you in this beautiful place.

(Note: Please pause after each question to allow the participant time to visualize and process.)

You see an animal standing in front of you:

1. What animal is it? . . . What is its size? . . . Its color?
2. What is your overall impression of this animal?
3. Now become the animal.
4. Experience your animal body and how you feel being in it.
5. What are your qualities? . . . And what can you do as this animal?
6. How do you feel being this animal?
7. Look around and view your environment. Where are you?
8. What do you see? What do you smell? What do you hear? And what do you sense?
9. You might see other animals that you can interact with . . .
10. Have a spontaneous experience now, doing whatever you choose . . . *(Give extra time)*
11. What qualities would you like to bring back with you? And how will this improve your life?
12. Now, thank the animal for allowing you to experience it.

And become yourself again . . . knowing that you can always reconnect and communicate with this animal whenever you choose . . .

And now, begin to focus your attention on the outside world, as you hear the sounds around you . . . Feel the surface under you . . . Feeling comfortable and content, focused and refreshed. Remembering everything you saw and experienced . . . Feeling relaxed, re-centered, and rejuvenated. Stretching your fingers and toes, counting up one and two peaceful and content as you return to awareness . . . More aware and alert, three and four . . . And, as I say . . . the number five . . . slowly opening your eyes.

HAVE AN ADVENTURE AS AN ANIMAL

PURPOSE: *SELF-DISCOVERY*

SUMMARY: Become an animal and have a spontaneous adventure as the animal. Receive a somatic message through it. *Note: After the participant has discussed their personal interpretation about their experience, you can look up the animal in the Quick Reference USD (Universal Symbol Dictionary) for more information about its qualities.*

MY EXPERIENCE: This is a light, fun imagery to use with groups and individuals. It's also a great icebreaker for a newly formed group or those who have never done imagery before.

EXAMPLE: Chris visualized a beautiful, strong horse that was made of blue light. The horse reared up on its hind legs and became "electric." Instead of fearing the horse, Chris was in awe of it. When he became it, he felt its energy and power. He said it gave him a message that there was nothing to fear, that there was health and energy ahead of him. Chris said it was an amazing experience that reassured him about his future.

ANIMAL ADVENTURE: INSIGHT PAGE QUESTIONS

1. Describe the animal you saw.
2. What was its size? Its color?
3. How did it feel to be the animal? What did you like about it?
4. What qualities did you have as the animal?
5. What were your capabilities as the animal?
6. If you had a name as the animal, what was your name?
7. What spontaneous adventure did you have?
8. How did it feel? And what does this mean to you?
9. Did you receive any other information or insight from being the animal?
10. If so, what was it? And how can you use it in your life?

ANIMAL AS HEALTH AND SOBRIETY

"Some people talk to animals. Not many listen though . . ."~ A.A. Milne

Closing your eyes now . . . Giving yourself permission to completely relax . . . Letting go of all muscles from head to toe . . . As you release all thoughts and things . . . Any sounds you hear, relaxing more deeply . . . Sinking into the surface you're on . . . Relaxing into the quiet, calm contentment of the imagination . . . Relaxing deeper with each breath you take, each beat of your heart, each word you hear . . . And even . . . the spaces . . . between my words . . . Becoming aware that you're in the most beautiful open field, with green grass swaying from left to right, and right to left . . . You smell the fresh, pungent aroma of the earth . . . Breathe in the air of the perfect temperature . . . Look out at the small lake in front of you . . . As the sun sparkles off the water like diamonds . . . hear the lake lapping slowly against the shore . . . In that timeless way . . . You are so relaxed . . . as you hear the leaves of the trees . . . rustle in the breeze . . .

And now, in this peaceful place, you see an animal that represents health and sobriety standing in front of you.

(Note: Please pause after every question to allow the participant time to visualize and process.)

1. What animal is it?.
2. Notice its size and its color . . . Notice its qualities.
3. What is your impression of this animal?
4. What does this animal think of you?
5. What do you like about it?
6. You find that you have a gift for the animal. What is the gift?
7. And now, the animal has a gift for you. What is this gift?
8. Now the animal gives you a message regarding sobriety.
9. Listen . . . you might hear the answer, or just intuitively know what the answer is.
10. Now, if you choose, become the animal, and feel that feeling of health and sobriety. As the animal, look at yourself (the person). What do you think of this person? Is there anything you'd like to say to them?

Becoming yourself again . . . Thank the animal in whatever way you choose for the information it brought, knowing you can always speak to this animal again whenever you choose.

And now, beginning to return to room consciousness. Feeling more aware as you hear my words and the sounds in and outside. With each word I say and each breath you take in and release, becoming more aware. Beginning to stretch your arms and legs and taking in an invigorating breath, feeling more alert and refreshed from this journey within. Remembering everything you saw and experienced clearly . . . And now, feeling rejuvenated and revitalized and ready for the rest of the day . . . as you open your eyes . . . to the light of the room . . .

<u>BELIEFS ABOUT SOBRIETY (OR OTHER ISSUE)</u>

PURPOSE: *ADDICTION, SOBRIETY*

SUMMARY: Participant and animal exchange gifts needed for sobriety. Participant receives a message from the animal regarding sobriety. The participant may choose to become the animal to *experience* it.

MY EXPERIENCE: Participants often cry insightful or joyful tears with this imagery. The messages from the animal can range from "The deer told me to be gentle with myself" to "Stop lying! Be honest about how you feel!"

EXAMPLE: Frank sees a wolf that represents sobriety. He's surprised, as he has no attachment to wolves. He says, "The wolf was very intelligent and seemed kind of dangerous. It knew me very well. I knew I had to be careful with it. I couldn't be aggressive or overly confident, or it could bite me." After considering this, Frank says, "I think this means I have to respect sobriety to keep it. I can't play games with it, or myself. I have to be honest."

ADAPTATION: As with the Animal Representing imagery, this one can be adapted to almost any issue, emotion, quality, or condition: love, success, courage, surrender, patience, acceptance, etc.

ANIMAL AS HEALTH AND SOBRIETY: INSIGHT PAGE QUESTIONS

1. What animal came to you to represent health and sobriety?
2. Describe the animal: its size, color, condition, attributes, and anything that stood out.
3. What did you think of the animal? What did it think of you?
4. How did you feel being near it?
5. What gift did you give the animal for health and sobriety?
6. What did the animal give you for continued health and sobriety?
7. What was its message regarding health and sobriety?
8. If you became the animal, how did it feel?
9. What did you (as the animal) think of you (the person)? And what message did you (the animal) give you (the person)? And what does this mean to you?
10. How can you best use this information for health and sobriety?

ANIMAL REPRESENTING . . .

"Animals are such agreeable friends—they ask no questions, they pass no criticisms." ~ George Eliot

With this imagery, choose an emotion, issue, or quality you want to address, such as love, joy, compassion, sadness, fear, anger, addiction, transition, decision, acceptance, courage, loyalty, etc.

Relaxing into the surface you're on . . . Allowing your body to relax into gravity . . . Closing your eyes as you're ready . . . Taking in a deep, healing breath as you allow all your muscles to expand and let go, slowing down by taking another healing breath and releasing that. Gently breathing into your stomach and up into your chest . . . and exhaling . . . with complete permission to relax and rest . . . into the stillness of the moment, into your center, in the here and now. Breathing in and out . . . and out and in . . . as breathing becomes slower and deeper . . . and rhythmic . . . And you shift your attention inward into the imagination . . . Where you find yourself standing in front of a small lake . . . that glitters under the sun . . . You smell the fresh, clean smell of earth and hear the trees gently rustling in the breeze . . .

And now you see an animal that represents (emotion, issue, or quality).

(Note: Please pause after each question to allow the participant time to visualize and process.)

1. What animal is it? Look at its size and its color.
2. Notice its qualities.
3. What is your impression of this animal?
4. What condition is it in?
5. What does this animal think of you?
6. What do you like about it? And dislike?
7. And now, become the animal.
8. What do you experience as the animal?
9. And as the animal, what do you think of you, the person?
10. And now, become yourself again.
11. The animal has a message for you. Just listen: you might hear it or intuitively know what the message is.

Thank the animal in whatever way you choose for the information it brought.

And now, beginning to focus your attention on the outside world again, as you hear the sounds around you . . . Feeling the surface under you . . . Feeling comfortable and content, focused and refreshed. Remembering everything you saw and experienced . . . Beginning to stretch your fingers and toes, counting up one and two . . . Feeling peaceful and content as you return to awareness . . . More aware and alert, three . . . and four . . . And on the count of five, opening your eyes to the light of the room, refreshed, relaxed, and aware . . .

DIALOGUE WITH ANIMAL ABOUT EMOTION, ISSUE, OR QUALITY

PURPOSE: *CLARITY*

SUMMARY: Participant visualizes an animal. They have a dialogue, receive a message, and become the animal, to experience greater understanding.

MY EXPERIENCE: Even those who aren't animal lovers feel safe as they connect to animals within imagery. I often witness people visualizing animals that they are very unfamiliar with, and are surprised to see, but there's always an important factor in why this particular animal shows up to give the person a message.

EXAMPLE: Ashly sees a large, silly bear that represents fear, which she finds surprising and a bit comical. Becoming the bear gives Ashly a feeling of strength and a feeling of levity at the irony. She receives the message, "It's okay! Even bears get scared! You're stronger than you know." Ashly later says this reminds her that she's strong and inspires her to move through fear.

ADAPTATION: Any emotion, issue, or quality can be used with this animal imagery for self-discovery: fear, joy, resentment, gratitude, acceptance, health, codependency, love, independence, hope, etc.

ANIMAL REPRESENTING: INSIGHT PAGE QUESTIONS

1. What animal came to you to represent your (emotion, quality, person, or challenge)?
2. Describe its qualities: appearance . . . size . . . color . . . condition . . . attitude.
3. What did you sense about this animal?
4. How did it feel being near it? What did you like about it?
5. Was there anything you disliked about it?
6. What did it think of you?
7. If you became the animal, how did it feel?
8. As the animal, what did you think of you, the person?
9. What was its message regarding your issue or situation?
10. And what does this mean to you?
11. How can you best use this information in your present life?

ANIMALS AS PARENTS

*"Perhaps there is a soul hidden in everything and it can always speak,
without even making a sound, to another soul." ~ Frances Hodgson Burnett*

Relax into the surface you're on and feel how you're completely supported . . . Close your eyes as you inhale peace and calm, and exhale anything unlike it . . . And as I count down from five to one, find yourself becoming deeply relaxed into the peaceful rhythm of the present . . . Counting down five and four, down three and two, deeper into relaxation, and all the way down to one . . . very relaxed . . . Journeying inward . . . into the imagination . . . You are standing in an open field of golden grass on the most beautiful day . . . Nothing but the flaxen field around you and a bright blue sky above you . . . as far as you can see. You breathe in the sweet, clean fragrance of the earth and hear the grass rustling in the gentle breeze. It slowly sways from left to right, and right to left. The soft warmth of the sun soothes you, and all the subtle sensations of this peaceful place . . . take you deeper into the imagination, where anything is possible . . .

(Note: Please pause after each question to allow the participant to visualize and process.)

FATHER

And now you see an animal that represents your father standing in front of you.

1. What animal is it?
2. Notice its size, its color, and what condition it's in.
3. What is your overall impression of this animal?
4. What do you like about it? And dislike?

Become the animal now and look back at yourself. How do you, as the animal, feel about you, the person? And what would you like to say to you, the person? Become yourself again.

MOTHER

And now you see an animal that represents your mother standing in front of you.

1. What animal is it?
2. Notice its size, its color, and what condition it's in.
3. What is your overall impression of the animal?
4. What do you like about it? And dislike?

Become the animal and look back at yourself. As the animal, how do you feel about you, the person? And what would you like to say to you, the person? Now become yourself again.

INTERACTION

Now, the animal that represents your father and the animal that represents your mother observe one another. Just allow them to have a spontaneous experience and watch. How do they respond to one another? What happens? And how do you feel about that? And now they give you a message. Listen to what they have to say.

And now, remembering everything you saw and experienced, coming back into the room refreshed and renewed, as I count up from one to five. Counting up one and two, hearing my voice . . . and the sounds inside the room. Becoming aware of your breath, and your body. Counting up three and four . . . beginning to stretch your arms and your legs . . . and counting up . . . relaxed and revitalized . . . opening your eyes on the count of . . . five.

FAMILY DYNAMICS

PURPOSE: *RELATIONSHIPS, FAMILY*

SUMMARY: Participant meets two animals representing parents and converses with them separately. Then the two animals have a spontaneous interaction and give the participant a message.

MY EXPERIENCE: I have often had clients say, after experiencing this, "I want to talk to my mother (or father) about this imagery." If one or both parents are unavailable to speak with, it can be therapeutic to write a letter to one or the other about the feelings the imagery elicits.

EXAMPLE: April sees a deer that represents her father. She likes her father's gentleness but doesn't like his passivity. Her father's message is, "I love you." She sees a tiger representing her mother. She likes the tiger's strength and doesn't like its aggression. The tiger's message is, "I've needed to be strong." The animals as parents together give her the message, "We can each love you in our own way." The animals walk off in different directions with no interaction. April affirms that her parents rarely speak, which saddens her. She says the message she receives from the animals lightens her heart, as it confirms what she knows is true: that they both love her, though they're not together.

ADAPTATION: You can substitute siblings, grandparents, close friends, etc.

ANIMALS AS PARENTS: INSIGHT PAGE QUESTIONS

Note: Ask these questions first for father, then for mother.

FATHER/MOTHER

1. Describe the animal that represented your father/mother.
2. What size was it? What was its color?
3. What condition was it in? What did you sense about it?
4. What did you like about it? And what didn't you like?
5. How did the animal feel about you?
6. How did it feel if you became the animal? And what did you say to you, the person?
7. What message did the animal give you?
8. And how can you use this in your life?

INTERACTION

1. How did the animals representing your mother and father interact?
2. How did you feel about their interaction?
3. What message did they give to you together? And how can you use this message to better your life?

ANIMALS HEAD AND STOMACH

"Feel your way into the thought rather than thinking your way into the feeling." ~ Abraham Hicks

Close your eyes as you allow your entire body to relax . . . Feel how the surface you're on supports you completely . . . allowing all muscles in your body to relax into gravity. Feeling so relaxed and finding that you're now in the most beautiful green meadow. You smell the fresh scent of earth and see a small lake in front of you. The sun shimmers off the water as it moves rhythmically toward shore . . . You hear it lap against the shore in that timeless way that seems to go on forever . . . A breeze of the perfect temperature moves over you. Feeling safe and sound as you enjoy this moment of complete peace . . . and moving into the imagination now . . . where everything is possible . . . (pause).

And now the most interesting thing happens. You feel a scratching from the inside of the top of your head, and you realize that there's an animal that wants to get out of your head. Just allow it to pop out of your head—and there it is, standing in front of you.

(Note: Please pause after every question to allow the participant time to visualize and process.)

1. What animal is it?
2. Notice its size, its color, and the condition it's in.
3. What is your impression of this animal?
4. What do you like about it? And dislike?
5. And what does this animal think of you?
6. Become the animal. *(Give ample time)*
7. How did it feel to be this animal? Now become yourself again.
8. The animal has a message for you now. Just listen . . . You might hear it or just know it intuitively. Thank the animals for the information they brought.

And now you feel a scratching from the inside of your stomach. And you realize that there's an animal that wants to get out of your stomach. Just allow it to pop out of your stomach. And there it is, standing in front of you.

1. What animal is it?
2. Notice its size, its color, its qualities, and the condition it's in.
3. What is your impression of this animal?
4. What do you like about it? And dislike?
5. And what does this animal think of you?
6. Become the animal. *(Give ample time)*
7. How does it feel to be this animal? Now become yourself again.
8. The animal now has a message for you. Just listen . . . you might hear the message or just know it intuitively.

Now, the animals from your head and your stomach notice one another. Allow them to have a spontaneous experience and watch what they do.

And now, returning . . . Remembering everything you saw and experienced clearly . . . As I begin to count up from one to five . . . Counting up one . . . And two . . . Feeling more alert . . . Relaxed and refreshed from this journey within . . . Bringing all messages back with you . . . Up three and four . . . Beginning to stretch your fingers and toes . . . Feeling refreshed . . . And opening your eyes on the count of . . . five.

REVEALS THOUGHTS AND EMOTIONS

PURPOSE: *SELF-AWARENESS*

SUMMARY: See an animal from the head (thinking) and an animal from the stomach (feeling). Qualities, attitude, condition, behavior, and the messages from the two animals give information regarding current thoughts and emotions and their interplay. Do the animals play together, or are they natural prey in the wild? Does one animal attack or eat the other? If so, which one? *Note: After the imagery and discussion of what these animals mean to the participant, you can look animals up in the Universal Symbol Dictionary for other qualities they might possess.*

MY EXPERIENCE: Clients are always amazed at how this imagery reveals or confirms what's going on with their thoughts and emotions. It's a great imagery to discover the subconscious mind's wisdom and valuable insight.

EXAMPLE: Kaetlyn sees a squirrel from her head. The squirrel darts from side to side, then stops and stares into her eyes and says, "Slow down!" She then sees a dolphin from her stomach, which she relates to as "playful, intelligent, and happy." The dolphin's message is "Let's have fun!" The squirrel jumps on the dolphin's back and smiles. The dolphin takes the happy squirrel for a ride through the water. Kaetlyn says she enjoyed this because fun and excitement have been lacking in her life recently. She comments that she needs to create a balance between work and fun.

ANIMALS HEAD AND STOMACH: INSIGHT PAGE QUESTIONS

Note: Please ask these questions first for the animal from the head, then from the stomach.

1. What animal came from your head/stomach?
2. What size was it? And it's color?
3. What condition was it in? What was your overall impression of this animal?
4. What did you like about it? Or dislike?
5. What did it think of you?
6. How did you feel when (if) you became it?
7. What was its message?
8. And what does this mean to you?

INTERACTION

1. How did the animals from your head and stomach respond to one another?
2. What did you notice about their interaction?
3. What does this mean to you and how can you use it to improve your life?

BACKPACK

*"Sometimes you don't realize the weight of a burden you've been carrying
until you feel the weight of its release." ~Anonymous*

Relax into the surface you're on . . . Take in a deep relaxation breath . . . Down into your stomach . . . And up into your chest . . . Letting that go, along with all the day's thoughts and concerns, anything that isn't right here and right now. Allowing all the muscles in your body to relax from your head down through your hands and into your feet. Getting very comfortable . . . enjoying this moment of peace and quiet . . . Continue breathing in and out, in and out, as you begin to journey inward to your imagination. And you find that . . .

You are walking along a desert path. The land and sky stretch out to the horizon. Breathe in the warm, still air. Notice any scents. The temperature is so comfortable. Feel the warmth of the sun on your body. Look out at the vast desert and sky. As you continue to walk, you notice that you have a backpack on. You feel the heaviness of the pack on your shoulders.

(Note: Please pause after every question to allow the participant time to visualize and process.)

1. What is the size of the backpack?
2. What is its weight and how does it feel?

You realize that there is something in the backpack that has been weighing you down. Up ahead, you see a smooth flat rock that you can sit on, and you decide to take a rest. You instinctively know what the heaviness in the backpack is.

3. What is it?

Take the backpack off, open it up, and find the heavy item. Take it out and take some time to observe it.

4. Now ask it what its purpose was.
5. Thank it for whatever it did for you. And if you choose to leave it behind, tell it why you no longer need to carry it.
6. Say goodbye to it in whatever way you choose.

Now put the backpack on again and continue on your walk. How does it feel without that unneeded item?

And now, beginning to return to room consciousness . . . Beginning to become more aware as you pay attention to your breath . . . Hearing my words and the sounds in and outside . . . With each word I say . . . And each breath you take in . . . And release . . . Becoming more aware of the outer world. Stretching your arms and legs as you take in a refreshing breath, feeling more alert . . . Hearing the sound of my voice and remembering everything you saw and experienced. Wiggling your fingers and toes . . . And now, gently, opening your eyes . . . rejuvenated and revitalized . . . and ready for the rest of the day.

<u>CHOOSE WHETHER TO RELEASE A BURDEN</u>

PURPOSE: *RELEASE, SELF-CARE*

SUMMARY: Take off a heavy backpack while hiking, remove the heavy object from it, and dialogue with it. Identify what you have been carrying and decide if it's time to release it or not.

MY EXPERIENCE: This imagery is short and to-the-point. Clients usually easily identify what the weight they're carrying is and feel to what extent it limits them. They also get in touch with how willing they are to release it.

EXAMPLE: Within the imagery, Katie feels excessive weight in the backpack that makes it difficult to walk. She feels overwhelmed carrying it and also barely remembers being without it. She pulls out a large, heavy stone from the backpack. She says it represents addiction, and she feels reticent to leave it, but says, "I know I can't keep carrying it. I have to leave it behind, or I won't make it."

ADAPTATION: The backpack can go unnamed (as in its present format), or it can be named to represent any issue: the backpack of anger, resentment, fear, protection, indecision, codependency, addiction, etc.

BACKPACK: INSIGHT PAGE QUESTIONS

1. How did you feel walking through the desert?
2. Describe your backpack.
3. What was its weight? And how did you feel carrying it?
4. What was the item/situation that weighed you down? How did it look?
5. What was its purpose?
6. Did you feel you still needed it?
7. If not, why do you no longer need to carry it?
8. If you decided to leave it behind, how did you say goodbye to it?
9. If you removed it from the backpack, how did you feel walking without it?
10. What will this allow you to do moving forward?

BIRD

"There is freedom waiting for you, on the breezes of the sky, and you ask,
'What if I fall?' Oh but my darling, what if you fly?" ~ Erin Hanson

Take in a deep relaxation breath, letting all your muscles from head to toe open up, loosen, and relax... Allowing your body to completely let go, with each breath you take in and release... along with all the day's thoughts and concerns... So completely supported... as you shift your attention into the soothing center of stillness. Where subtle signs of deep relaxation allow all the muscles in your body to relax so deeply... drifting inward... into the world of the imagination... where all is possible...

And now, imagine that you are a bird. Take a few moments to feel your bird body and realize what kind of bird you are.

(Note: Please pause after each question to allow the participant time to visualize and process.)

1. Notice your size . . . and color(s) . . . your eyes . . . beak . . . body . . . and wings.
2. What are your qualities as this bird?
3. Look around as the bird. Where are you? You can choose to stay just where you are, or you can move around in your bird body.
4. How does it feel being this bird?

Look around as your bird-self and view the landscape you're in. Feel the breeze, notice the sky. Notice the scents you smell. And knowing that you have the ability to fly, open your wings and feel the air lift you up easily and naturally. You spread your wings in a natural rhythm . . . and rest upon the air . . . you can float and glide . . . Enjoying the scenery below, flying wherever you choose, over land or water, seeing life from a bigger perspective. Enjoying this freedom and the amazing ability of your imagination to take you anywhere. (ample pause) And now, becoming yourself again, with the freedom of that bird within you.

You are free to stretch your imagination, free to stretch your beliefs, to make them real through action. Just like the people who first flew, people like you, who bypassed disbelief and made dreams come true, you are able and capable, and your imagination is taking you there.

1. What vision or goal do you choose to stretch your thinking towards?
2. What qualities can you expand to make it possible?
3. What is it you *will* do once you believe it is possible?
4. Imagine yourself doing that now.

You see yourself doing what you want... Focusing in on the scene... The colors... The brightness... And the clarity... Your smile... The activities. You see and feel your success, reaping all the good feelings and gratification that come from fulfilling your dream. Because *you chose* to stretch your thoughts and beliefs... into actions.

And now, beginning to return... remembering everything you saw and experienced clearly... Counting up one and two. Feeling more alert and inspired from this journey within... Up three and four... Feeling the surface under you, grounded and supported. Stretching your fingers and toes... And opening your eyes on the count of five, renewed... revitalized... and ready for the rest of the day.

EXPERIENCE A GOAL AS ACCOMPLISHED

PURPOSE: *CONFIDENCE*

SUMMARY: Become a bird, fly above the earth, and stretch the imagination. Clearly re-imagine a dream as possible and successful. The participant imagines feeling and experiencing all the benefits received. *Note: You can look up additional qualities of the bird in the Universal Symbol Dictionary after personal meanings of the bird are discussed with participant.*

MY EXPERIENCE: Some people will become the bird and never fly but still receive valuable information through the bird's qualities.

EXAMPLE: Roland wants to open his own business. He has skills that could make a business work, but he finds it hard to believe in himself. Within the imagery, he becomes a falcon. He feels the sense of rising above, having a wide and clear vision. He remembers his grandfather saying that, "Falcons are tenacious." In the imagery he sees the grand opening of his business: people congratulating him, his customers and finances increasing with time. It feels real, giving him hope and inspiration.

BIRD: INSIGHT PAGE QUESTIONS

1. What kind of bird were you?
2. What size and what color(s) were you? Describe your eyes, beak, wings. Was there anything that stood out about the bird?
3. Describe how it felt being this bird. What are the bird's qualities?
4. How did it feel flying above the earth? What did you see as you flew?
5. What situation or qualities did you choose to expand?
6. How did it feel to expand your thoughts, ideas, and abilities?
7. And how did it feel to be successful and gratified?
8. What is the first step, or the next step you can take to make this vision reality?

BRIDGE ACROSS THE RIVER

"The deeper that sorrow carves into your being, the more joy you can contain." ~Khalil Gibran

Feel how you are supported completely by the surface you're on. A wave of deep relaxation moves down through your head behind your forehead and eyes. All muscles soften, relaxing from your head to toes. Going deeper . . . relaxed . . . as I count down five and four, three and two, deeper and deeper relaxed, through the neck, shoulders, arms. Down your torso and through your legs. And all the way down to one. You now see that you're standing in a heavenly green meadow. There is a small river flowing through it, like a ribbon of light under the sun. The temperature is perfect under the expansive blue sky. A breeze moves over your skin, and you smell the fresh aroma of the earth. There is a beautiful, strong tree across the river, and a bridge leading to it.

And now, invite a wise, all-loving, compassionate guide to join you in this beautiful place.

(Note: Please pause after each question to allow the participant time to visualize and process.)

1. Allow your guide to appear in front of you.
2. Feel their qualities of pure love and compassion. Ask your guide their name.
3. Greet them in whatever way you choose.
4. Your guide points you toward the bridge that leads across the river. You begin walking toward the bridge and over the bridge. You see a beautiful tree ahead of you. As you arrive at the tree, feel the complete silence and serenity.
5. Now a person you have loved very much appears under the tree. Who is this, and how do they appear?
6. Notice the look in their eyes.
7. Greet them in whatever way you choose.
8. Say whatever you need to say to them.
9. How do they respond?
10. Is there anything you'd like to ask them? If so, do that now.
11. How do they respond?
12. How does your guide respond to this?
13. Enjoy the presence of this person and say whatever else is needed.
14. Ask them what they want for you and listen to their answer.

Knowing this person lives in your heart always and lives through you in many ways, thank them for what they gave you. Say goodbye, knowing that you can speak to them again whenever you choose. Now thank your guide, knowing they are always there when called upon.

And now, becoming more aware of my voice and the room around you . . . Remembering everything you saw and experienced, beginning to come back to room awareness, as I count up from one to five. Counting up one . . . And two . . . Hearing my voice . . . Hearing sounds in and outside the room . . . Feeling the surface under you . . . Feeling centered and grounded . . . Counting up three . . . and four . . . beginning to stretch your arms . . . Refreshed and revitalized and counting to five . . . opening your eyes to the light of the room.

DIALOGUE WITH A SEPARATED LOVED ONE

PURPOSE: *GRIEF, INSPIRATION*

SUMMARY: Meet a guide for support, and then together meet with a loved one from whom you are separated by life transition or death. Have the opportunity to speak with the loved one to ask questions, as well as receive information. *Note: Participants often cry during this imagery, receive connection, and find some closure with a loved one.*

MY EXPERIENCE: This is a poignant, emotional imagery. Clients often cry with sadness and/ or joy as they connect with their loved one. Just as people respond individually to grief, this imagery brings up what clients are ready to deal with. There is sometimes anger, which when released, leads to greater love, forgiveness, and a greater sense of understanding.

EXAMPLE: Stephanie's father died two years ago, and she's missing his presence and guidance in her life. She is single and feeling isolated. She meets her guide, who is Jesus. They walk across the river together. She and her father greet with hugs, he tells her that he's very happy. He says he's proud of her and that he just wants her to be happy. He suggests that she "go out and live life." Jesus and Stephanie walk back across the river. Stephanie states that, "It felt so real!" and says, "I know it's time for me to start living again."

BRIDGE ACROSS THE RIVER: INSIGHT PAGE QUESTIONS

1. Describe your guide. What were the qualities of your guide? What was your guide's name?
2. Whom did you see across the river, under the tree?
3. How did you feel seeing this person?
4. Describe how they looked/felt.
5. How did they respond to you?
6. What did you say to them? And what was the response?
7. What did this person say they want for you?
8. How did you respond?
9. How did you say goodbye?
10. How did it feel to connect with this person? How can you use the information they gave you?

CANYON

"Obstacles don't have to stop you. If you run into a wall, don't turn around and give up.
Figure out how to climb it, go through it, or work around it." ~ Michael Jordan

Closing your eyes as you get settled into the surface you're on . . . Taking in a long, deep healing breath, inhaling from your stomach up into your chest, and releasing it as you let go of all of the day's thoughts and concerns . . . Drifting down into a soothing state of serenity . . . Taking in another deep healing breath . . . into the stomach . . . And exhaling anything unlike peace and serenity . . . Feeling centered, soothed, and content . . . As you rest into the stillness . . . Drifting deeper . . . Into relaxation. Into the imagination . . . And now . . .

(Note: Please pause after each question to allow the participant time to visualize and process.)

Think of a goal that you want to accomplish and might be having difficulty with. Whatever it is, imagine a symbol that represents this goal when completed and realized.

1. See the symbol clearly in your mind. Observe its size . . . shape . . . color . . . and the feeling of the symbol.

And now see that you are walking through a beautiful canyon with towering rocks on each side of you. You know that at the end of this canyon is that symbol representing your goal realized. As you walk on the path, you see distinct colors and designs in the rocks. You feel the warmth of the sun coming down in shafts of light. You absorb the silence that surrounds you. The air is dry and still, and the sky is a vivid blue. The canyon path widens and narrows as it weaves through the wall of rocks on each side.

2. As it tapers and winds to the right, you turn the corner to see a rock blocking the path. This rock represents a quality or attitude that is keeping you from your goal. What is that quality or attitude?
3. You know instinctively that there is a way for you to continue forward. And you know that there is a tool to get you past it. What is it that will help you continue past this challenge?
4. There is always a way. You look around you, and you see a tool that represents overcoming your challenge. What kind of tool is it?
5. Now use the tool to clear your path. You are past the block now—the path is wide open. You see the symbol of the completion of your goal ahead of you.
6. And now you reach the symbol. Step into the symbol and experience the feeling of your goal completed.

See yourself enjoying the completion of your goal. Notice the benefits and how you feel. See the colors, the details and any benefits others receive.

And now, feeling more aware as you prepare to come back to room consciousness . . . Hearing my words and the sounds in and outside of the room. Beginning to stretch your arms and legs . . . Taking in a refreshing breath of air. Oxygenating your body. Feeling rejuvenated from this journey within. Remembering everything you saw and experienced clearly. Becoming more alert as you stretch your body and open your eyes, revitalized, renewed, and ready for the rest of the day.

OVERCOME OBSTACLE TO ATTAIN GOAL

PURPOSE: *MOTIVATION*

SUMMARY: Walk through a canyon toward an unrealized goal and come across an obstacle. Discover how much power you are giving this obstacle. Grasp the quality or action (as a tool) that will help you to move through or remove this obstacle. Recognize the next step to take toward reaching your goal.

MY EXPERIENCE: This is a good imagery to bring insight to clients who feel stuck in attaining a goal, even a goal they might not know they have.

EXAMPLE: Hassan moved far from his childhood home. He feels homesick and vulnerable having just a few new friends. His goal is to feel more at home in his new city. Within the imagery, the tool he found to clear his path was a phone. He realized that the phone represented communication, and that he was the one who wasn't reaching out to the new friends he'd met, thinking they would judge him when he's not at his best. After reaching out to a new friend, he and his friend found that they have many interests and values in common. He expressed that his new friend really appreciates him for who he is. He's feeling better about his move now and ready to create more friendships and make this new city his home.

CANYON: INSIGHT PAGE QUESTIONS

1. What goal did you focus on? Was it the goal you *thought* you would focus on?
2. What makes this goal important to you?
3. Describe the symbol that you saw that represented your successful completion of the goal.
4. What obstacle (attitude, situation, belief) did it represent in your present life?
5. What size was the obstacle in your path?
6. What was the tool that helped you overcome the block?
7. What attribute or attitude does the tool represent?
8. How did you overcome the obstacle?
9. Was it easy or difficult to get past it?
10. With the path clear, how did it feel reaching your goal?
11. How did it feel when you became one with the symbol representing your desire?
12. How can you use this information now to take action on your desire?

CAR

"Logic will get you from A to B. Imagination will take you anywhere." ~ Albert Einstein

Settle into the surface you're on . . . And let your body relax into gravity. Close your eyes as you're ready. Take in a deep relaxation breath as you allow all your muscles to expand and let go, as you slow down by taking another relaxation breath in and releasing it. Gently breathe into your stomach and up into your chest and exhale. Give yourself complete permission to relax and rest into the stillness of the moment. Relax into your center, in the here and now. Breathing in and out, and out and in, as your breathing becomes slower and deeper . . . And you shift your attention inward, into the center of calm and contentment within you. Your mind and body at peace, as you move deeper into that center to allow yourself to wonder and wander . . . into your imagination . . . you find that . . .

You're in a vehicle driving on a road representing (subject of the imagery: joy, love, pain, addiction, etc.).

(Note: Please pause at each step and allow the participant to visualize and process.)

1. What is the condition of the road?
2. And how does it feel driving on it?
3. Notice the vehicle you're in. What color is it?
4. What shape?
5. What are the qualities of this car?
6. Describe the interior.
7. How does it feel driving this car? Are there any sounds you hear as you drive?
8. What do you like about it? Is there anything you'd like to change?
9. Look at the scenery as you drive past. What do you see out the windows?
10. In what direction are you headed?
11. Is the road straight, curvy, level, or going upward or downward?

Just allow yourself to experience the drive now. Feel the road under you and how the car maneuvers.

12. Do you know where you're going? . . . If you don't, how do you feel about that?
13. Now you arrive at a destination. Where are you?
14. How does it feel to be there? . . . And what do you plan to do now that you've arrived?

And now, begin to focus on the surface under you. As you hear the sounds around you . . . Feeling comfortable, content. Remembering everything you saw and experienced . . . Relaxed, calm, and centered. Beginning to stretch your fingers and toes, counting up one and two . . . feeling peaceful and focused as you return to awareness . . . More aware and alert, three and four . . . and beginning to open your eyes as I say . . . the number . . . five . . . and . . . opening your eyes . . . to the light of the room . . . refreshed, rejuvenated, and ready for the rest of the day.

DISCOVER VALUES, DESIRES, NEEDS

PURPOSE: *SELF-AWARENESS*

SUMMARY: The car represents the driver (self) and how they feel about their journey of (subject: relationships, career, sobriety, parenthood, independence, etc.) The car exemplifies the qualities they value or desire on their journey (comfort, beauty, prestige, strength, fun, adventure, speed). Note the qualities of the specific vehicle: Jeep/truck = outdoor adventures; sports car = speed, excitement; economy car = functionality; sedan = comfort, safety; SUV = family, adventure. *Note: The conditions of the car and road relate to the present level of ease or discomfort of the participant's journey. Ascending road = goals moving upward. Horizontal, level road = wanting or having a consistent foundation. Descending road = delving into the unknown, the subconscious, or "going downward" in mood or behavior. Use the USD to get information on further meanings of directions (south, north, east, west), colors, landscapes, and road texture and condition (smooth, rough, etc.)*

MY EXPERIENCE: This is a lighter, simpler imagery to use when emotionally impactful imagery isn't in order. It's also a good choice for group work and as an icebreaker.

EXAMPLE: Ruby envisioned herself driving up the California coast along the ocean. She was alone in a sports car with the top down on a perfect, sunny day. The car was white with a tan interior, which she said felt luxurious and comfortable. She felt free with all possibilities in front of her. She said, "The road was smooth, the scenery was beautiful, and I felt happy and excited about the future."

ADAPTATION: The car can represent different states of being: joy, anger, grief, solitude, loneliness, adventure, independence, confidence, focus, sobriety, etc.

CAR: INSIGHT PAGE QUESTIONS

1. What type of road were you on? What size was the road? What was the condition of the road?
2. What kind of vehicle were you driving?
3. In what direction were you headed? Describe the landscape you were driving through.
4. Was the road straight, curvy, level, on an incline or decline?
5. Did you know where you were headed? Was it important or not?
6. What color was the car? What condition was it in? How did the interior look and feel?
7. What did you like about this vehicle? And not like? Was there anything you'd change?
8. What did the vehicle represent to you?
9. As you arrived at your destination, what did you see there? And what did you plan to do next?

CAVERN

"Rock bottom is not your end; it is your beginning." ~ Christine Evangelou
"Job one is get out of that cave."~ Robert Downey Jr.

Getting comfortable now . . . Beginning to relax as I count down from five to one . . . Counting five . . . feeling more relaxed with each word . . . Down to four . . . More relaxed with each breath you take and release . . . More relaxed with each descending number . . . Down to three. Letting go of anything that isn't here and now. Counting down two . . . Another deep breath in and release . . . and . . . way down to one. Going into the imagination . . .

You're in a beautiful green meadow surrounded by trees and small hills. Colorful flowers are scattered throughout the grass; you watch them sway gently in the slight breeze. The meadow is fresh and alive with pleasing scents. There is one large, graceful tree near the edge of the meadow. You begin to walk toward this tree, and as you get close to it, you sense an energy. You realize that this tree is there just for you. There is a spiritual guide who loves you unconditionally that will meet you here. This guide wants only the very best for you. Invite your guide to join you here in this beautiful place.

(Note: Please pause after each question to allow the participant time to visualize and process.)

Your guide appears before you. What does your guide look like? How do you feel in their presence? Ask what name your guide would like to be called. Your guide now looks toward the small hill at the edge of the meadow. You see there is a large entrance to a cavern there. Your guide invites you to walk with them toward the cavern. You arrive at the entrance to the cavern, and see a path leading down into it. You begin walking down this path together, noticing the interesting sights on the way down.

Halfway down into the cavern, you realize that at the bottom of this cavern is The Room of (Issue: addiction, codependency, etc.). Your guide is taking you safely down to talk to (issue) for your benefit. Your guide is here to love, support, and protect you. You now arrive at the door of (issue). Open the door and walk in with your guide.

1. What do you see there?
2. How does (issue) look/represent itself?
3. And how do you feel being there with (issue)?
4. Your guide now says something to (issue) on your behalf. Just listen . . .
5. Tell (issue) what you were trying to get from it.
6. Inform it what it took from you.
7. And now tell (issue) how you are going to receive this in a healthier way in your life.
8. Say whatever else you want to say to (issue).
9. Say goodbye to (issue) in whatever way you choose.
10. Now close the door on (issue).

You and your guide begin walking up through the cavern, into the clean, fresh air of the meadow, and all possibilities. Thank your guide in whatever way you choose, knowing you can always call on them again.

Sit down now and rest under the beautiful tree. Look out at the field to watch the flowers sway gently in the breeze. Smell the fresh, clean scent of nature, feeling at one with it, safely grounded in the freedom of clarity.

And now, bringing back the calm and peace of nature, remembering everything you saw and experienced clearly . . . As I count up from one to five . . . Counting up one . . . and two . . . feeling more alert . . . relaxed and renewed . . . up three and four . . . Beginning to stretch your fingers and toes . . . Feeling more aware . . . And on the count of five . . . Opening your eyes . . . refreshed, revitalized, and ready for the rest of the day.

VISUALIZE AND DIALOGUE WITH ADDICTION

PURPOSE: *ADDICTION, SOBRIETY*

SUMMARY: Meet a guide for support who takes you into a cavern to dialogue with your issue (addiction, codependency, or any issue decided upon). Tell the issue what you were trying to get from it and what it took from you. Receive information from the issue and tell it how you plan to receive what you wanted from it in healthier ways. *Note: You can look in the Quick Reference USD for more information on the type of tree seen, as well as the visual (that symbolized the issue).*

MY EXPERIENCE: This is a very effective imagery to allow people to see or experience addiction (or other issues) in front of them so they can dialogue. The room of addiction (for example) can be anything from a pharmacy, a dark alley with needles, a bar, a bathroom, or the client as they appeared when using. Clients often feel wonderful when they walk up and out of the cavern. One client saw a window at the top of the cave and said, "It's so I can always look down on addiction to keep an eye on it from above."

EXAMPLE: Lauren is a twenty-one-year-old who has left rehab. She meets her guide, who is an angel named Maya. They go down into the cavern into the room of addiction. It is a small room with hundreds of bottles of pills. She feels frightened, but her guide, Maya, speaks to addiction, saying, "She won't be ruled by you anymore." Lauren tells addiction it took everything from her—relationships, family, and health—and that she now has sober friends, spiritual support, and tools to help her live a happy life.

ADAPTATION: This imagery can be adapted to any issue that you'd like to release or have more clarity about: addiction, habit, codependency, relationship, resentments, etc.

CAVERN INSIGHT PAGE QUESTIONS

1. Describe the tree you saw. What type of tree was it?
2. Describe your guide. What qualities did they possess?
3. What was your guide's name?
4. When you arrived at the room of (issue), what did (issue) look like?
5. Describe what you saw in the room.
6. How did you feel being there with it?
7. What did your guide say to (issue) on your behalf?
8. What did you tell your (issue) that you were trying to get from it?
9. What did you tell it that it took from you?
10. And how are going to receive that in a healthier way?

CHILD EXPECTED

"I loved you from the very start. You stole my breath, embraced my heart. Our life together has just begun. You're part of me, my little one." ~ Anonymous

Begin to settle into the surface you're on . . . getting as comfortable as you need to be. Letting your body relax into gravity . . . Closing your eyes as you're ready . . . Taking in a deep, relaxation breath as you allow all your muscles to expand and let go . . . Slowing down by taking in another relaxation breath and releasing it. Gently breathe into your stomach and up into your chest, and exhale. Giving yourself complete permission . . . to rest into the stillness of the moment. Relaxing into your center, in the here and now. Breathing in and out, and out and in, slower and deeper . . . Shifting your attention inward, into the center of calm and contentment within you. Mind and body at peace, moving deeper into that center . . . allowing yourself to wonder and wander . . . Drifting down to observe and absorb the quiet . . . in the center . . . of the soothing . . . silence . . . within.

You're in a beautiful, fertile valley, in the midst of an abundant meadow. Flowers blossom all around you, coming out of the lush, dark earth. As you sit on your blanket, on the greenest grass, you look up into a blue sky. The sun warms your face and body, and the air is fresh and life-giving. The green grass sways in the breeze. You feel safe and peaceful in this magical place.

(Note: Please pause after each question for the participant to visualize and process.)

1. Be aware of how it feels, anticipating the arrival of your child.
2. You relax and look around the meadow again. As you do, your child spontaneously appears sitting on the blanket beside you. What does your child look like?
3. How do you feel as you look at your child?
4. You look down to see that you have a gift for your child. What is the gift you give them?
5. What does it mean to you?
6. Now your child gives you a gift. What is this gift?
7. What does it look and feel like?
8. What does it mean to you?
9. Now your child looks into your eyes and has a message for you.
10. What is your child's message?
11. Now give your child a message. What do you want your child to know?
12. You lean over and embrace your child. How does this feel?
13. How does your child react?

Just enjoy this closeness for a moment. Knowing that this feeling can stay with you and you can access it any time you choose. Keeping your child within your heart until you see them before you.

And now, begin to focus your attention on the outside world again, as you hear the sounds around you . . . Feel the surface under you . . . Feeling comfortable and content, focused and refreshed. Remembering everything you saw and experienced . . . Feeling relaxed, re-centered, and rejuvenated. Beginning to stretch your fingers and toes, counting up one and two, feeling peaceful as you return to awareness . . . More aware and alert, three and four . . . And beginning to open your eyes, as I say . . . the number five . . . Feeling relaxed, refreshed, and ready for the rest of the day.

CONNECT WITH CHILD

PURPOSE: *RELATIONSHIPS, CHILD*

CAVEAT: This imagery should be used within an individual session (unless working with a group of expectant parents.) *Note:* Make sure you are well aware of the situation of the upcoming birth, adoption, etc. and that this imagery is appropriate.

SUMMARY: The purpose of this imagery is to connect with and feel love for the child you expect. Realize the gift you can give them and what gift they bring to you.

MY EXPERIENCE: This can be an exciting, inspirational, or moving imagery for those welcoming a child of any age. It is a great imagery to reconnect the expectant parent to the reality of the child's arrival into their life.

EXAMPLE: Paula is feeling excited about the upcoming birth of her child but uncertain about her relationship with the father. Within the imagery, she sees her child at six months of age, a beautiful boy with green eyes whom she feels overwhelming love for. The child gives her the gift of purpose, and she gives the child the gift of love and guidance. Within the imagery, the father remains in the scene, at a distance. Paula says, "He hasn't really tried to be a part of this, and I guess deep down I know I can't count on him." She has tears in her eyes as she says, "I can't wait to see my son."

CHILD EXPECTED: INSIGHT PAGE QUESTIONS

1. Describe your child.
2. How did it feel seeing and being with your child?
3. What gift did you have for your child?
4. What gift did your child have for you?
5. How did it feel embracing your child?
6. What did you tell your child?
7. What did your child tell you?
8. What was your overall feeling about this experience?
9. How can this information support you?

CHILDHOOD HOME

"There is nothing like returning to a place that remains unchanged
to find the ways in which you yourself have changed." ~ Nelson Mandela

Allowing yourself to get comfortable now . . . Closing your eyes when you're ready. Letting all your muscles open up . . . expand . . . and relax . . . Settling into the comfortable quiet of your breath. Noticing that there is a light of the most beautiful color surrounding your entire body. Taking in a healing breath, as you inhale peace and calm from this light. Feeling and seeing this healing light all around you. Inhaling peace . . . exhaling calm. Inhaling calm . . . exhaling peace. Absorbing peace and calm as you naturally breathe in the light surrounding you. Absorbing its healing properties, as it lights up your mind . . . moves down through your heart, brightening and glowing, down through your arms and into your hands . . . Down through your stomach, shimmering and sparkling, down through your abdomen . . . into your legs . . . Down into the bottom of your feet . . . Centered, content . . . and calm. And now you see that . . .

You are standing in front of your childhood home. Walk up to the door, turn the doorknob, and walk in.

(Note: Please pause at each step to allow the participant time to visualize and process.)

1. Begin walking around the house, looking at the different rooms.
2. What do you notice about this house that you didn't notice when you were younger?
3. Go to a special room in this house; take in the sights . . . the scents . . . and the feeling of the room. What makes this room special?
4. Now you notice a familiar item. Look carefully at this item. If you are able to pick it up, hold it and observe it. What is this item? And what does it mean to you?
5. What do you like about this home? What don't you like?
6. What did you learn about life in this home?
7. And how do you, or can you, use this lesson in your present life?
8. Now, you walk outside, to the back of the home, and you notice that someone from your past remains there. Who is it? *(pause)* How do you feel about this person?
9. Greet them and say whatever you feel you left unsaid. *(Give ample time.)*
10. If there is anything else you need to say, say it now.
11. How do they respond?
12. Thank them for whatever you learned from them.
13. Leave and look back at the home. If you want to change it, do that now, and say goodbye.

Beginning to become more aware of your surroundings now . . . the surface below you . . . as you prepare to come back. Becoming aware of sounds in and outside the room . . . And the sound of my voice . . . Aware of your breathing, relaxed and regular . . . Feeling lighter and more alert. Taking in a breath of energizing oxygen, coming back to room awareness, refreshed and rejuvenated, enlightened and at peace . . . As you open your eyes . . . to the light of the room . . .

VISIT YOUR CHILDHOOD HOME

PURPOSE: *CHILDHOOD ISSUES*

SUMMARY: Visit your childhood home. Realize what you learned there and how it can be used positively in your present life.

MY EXPERIENCE: This imagery is effective to empower clients through what they learned in their childhood home, whether the lessons came from supportive or challenging experiences. It also gives the client the opportunity to express what might have gone unsaid as a child. A good imagery to journal about.

EXAMPLE: Nickie saw a childhood home where she lived with her mother, brother, and stepfather during an unhappy time. She told her stepfather that she learned how not to treat a child from his behavior. She stated that she uses this lesson every day, as a mother, to positively nurture her own daughter.

CHILDHOOD HOME: INSIGHT PAGE QUESTIONS

1. How did you feel walking into this home?
2. What did you notice about it that you didn't notice when you were younger?
3. Was there a room that stood out to you? What makes this room special?
4. What was the familiar item you noticed? And what does it mean to you?
5. What do you like about this home? What don't you like?
6. Who did you see from the past?
7. How do you feel about this person? And what do they mean to you?
8. What did you tell them that you learned from them? And how did they respond?
9. What did you learn about life in this home?
10. How do you, or how *can* you, use this lesson in your present life?
11. Did you choose to change the home? If so, how did you change it?
12. And how did you say goodbye to the home?

CIRCLE OF SUPPORT

" If you have at least one person genuinely supporting you,
you're blessed." ~ Marc and Angel Chernoff

Begin to settle into the surface you're on . . . getting as comfortable as you need to be. Letting your body relax into gravity . . . Closing your eyes as you're ready . . . Taking in a deep relaxation breath as you allow all your muscles to expand and let go . . . Slowing down by taking in another relaxation breath and releasing it. Gently breathe into your stomach and up into your chest, and exhale. Giving yourself complete permission . . . to rest into the stillness of the moment. Relaxing into your center, in the here and now. Breathing in and out, and out and in, slower and deeper . . . Shifting your attention inward, into the center of calm and contentment within you. Mind and body at peace, moving deeper into that center . . . allowing yourself to wonder and wander . . . Drifting down to observe and absorb the quiet . . . in the center . . . of the soothing . . . silence . . . within.

You're in a beautiful opening of a pine forest. The air is fresh and cleansing. You're standing up on a pedestal in front of a circle of your loved ones. The people who truly love and support you are there to cheer you on. They have come to honor you for who you are and what you strive to be. They see and understand the deepest part of you. As you stand on this pedestal, you turn around the circle and see the faces of your loved ones. They smile, and you see the light of love shining through their eyes. They bow their heads slightly to you in recognition. Feel the love from them and send it back. They are here to remind you of who you are and what you are capable of.

(Note: Pause after questions to allow time for visualizing and processing.)

One old friend from childhood walks up to the microphone to tell the group of people what they love, admire, and appreciate about you.

1. Listen to what they say. You might hear it, or just know it intuitively. (longer pause)
2. And now a mentor, an older person whom you admire, steps up to tell the group what they love, admire and respect about you.
3. Listen to what they say. You might hear it, or just know it intuitively. (longer pause)

Now, the people in your circle of support form a line, each one coming to you, honoring you with words, a pat on the back, or an embrace. Feel the love and support this brings. Allow each person to tell you what they admire in you. Absorb this information, allowing you to remind yourself who you truly are and embody all that you are capable of.

Now bringing your attention back into the present. Remembering everything you saw and experienced . . . feeling calm, centered, and seen. Bringing back remembrances, feelings, and knowings . . . Breathing in a fresh breath of oxygen, vital and energizing . . . Beginning to move your fingers and toes . . . Stretching as you need . . . Feeling light and relaxed into the present . . . Being the gift of the present . . . as you open your eyes . . . calm, centered, and encouraged.

VERBAL SUPPORT THROUGH CELEBRATION

PURPOSE: *CONFIDENCE*

SUMMARY: Loved ones verbally support you. A childhood friend and an older mentor share what they love and admire about you. Your loved ones greet you in a line, tell you the pride they feel in you, and encourage you on your present journey.

MY EXPERIENCE: This imagery can be used for transitions, celebrations, successes, or challenging times when support is needed. It can provide reassurance, as well as empowerment and encouragement toward continued progress.

EXAMPLE: Brittany sees her loved ones around her: family, a childhood friend, and a mentor. She receives compliments on how much she's grown and how talented and loving she is. She cries softly during the ceremony and says how loved and inspired she feels.

CIRCLE OF SUPPORT: INSIGHT PAGE QUESTIONS

1. How did it feel being honored and supported by loved ones?
2. Who was the childhood friend that got up to speak about you?
3. What did they share about you?
4. Who was the older person/mentor who spoke about you?
5. And what did they say?
6. What did others say to you or express as they came to you?
7. What encouragement did you receive?
8. How can you use this support in your life at present?

COAT

"The best protection any woman can have is courage." ~ Elizabeth Cady Stanton

Getting settled into the surface you're on ... and closing your eyes. Taking in a long, deep healing breath. Inhaling from your stomach up into your chest and releasing it as you let go of all of the day's thoughts and concerns ... Drifting down into a soothing state of serenity ... Taking in another deep breath ... into the stomach ... and exhaling anything unlike peace and serenity ... Feeling centered, soothed, and content ... Breathing in one more deep healing breath ... into the stomach ... up into the chest and releasing it ... as you simply rest into the stillness. Your body and mind drifting deeper ... into relaxation ... all senses soothed. Drifting ... into the imagination.

You find you are walking down a street wearing a coat that represents protection.

(Note: Please pause after each question to allow participant time to visualize and process.)

1. What does the coat look like?
2. Of what material is it made?
3. What color or pattern is it?
4. What is its weight? ... How does it feel on your body?
5. As you walk down the street, how do you feel wearing this coat?
6. How do people respond to you?
7. What is this coat protecting you from?
8. You notice now that your coat has a pocket. You reach into the pocket and find a note regarding protection. Read its message.
9. You can choose to keep the coat or replace it with something else.
10. Or, you can simply choose to release it.
11. Whichever you decide to do, thank the coat for whatever it did, or does, for you.

And now, beginning to return to room consciousness ... Becoming more aware as you pay attention to your breath ... With each breath you take in ... and release ... becoming more aware of the outer world. Hearing my words ... and the sounds in and outside ... Beginning to stretch your arms and legs, taking in a refreshing breath, feeling more alert ... Remembering everything you saw and experienced. Wiggling your fingers and toes ... And now, gently, opening your eyes, rejuvenated and revitalized ... and ready for the rest of the day!

CHOOSE TO KEEP OR RELEASE PROTECTION

PURPOSE: *RELEASE*

SUMMARY: You wear a coat representing protection. You find a note inside the pocket with a message regarding protection. You choose to keep the coat, replace it with something else, or remove it.

MY EXPERIENCE: This imagery is effective in disclosing how willing a participant is to release a behavior or coping mechanism that might be limiting or unhealthy. They might also find that the protection is necessary and healthy for them. Protection can be emotional, physical, or mental.

EXAMPLE: Kai visualizes a heavy coat that "weighs her down." She says it reminds her of a coat she wore several years ago during a hard time in her life when her self-esteem was low and she was untrusting in relationships. She reaches inside the pocket and finds a note that says, "Improvement." She believes this means, "I'm beginning to trust my own judgment more, so I don't feel as over-protective of myself." She chooses to exchange the heavy coat for a lighter jacket.

ADAPTATION: This imagery can be adapted to any condition, emotion, issue, or quality to be released, such as a coat of anger, resentment, pride, codependency, addiction, etc.

COAT: INSIGHT PAGE QUESTIONS

1. Describe the coat you were wearing, including its material, design, and color.
2. What was its weight? How did it feel wearing the coat?
3. How did people respond to you (if they did)?
4. What was the coat protecting you from?
5. What message did the note give you?
6. How does that relate to protection in your present life?
7. Did you choose to keep the coat? If so, why?
8. If you removed it, describe how you ceremoniously did this.
9. If you exchanged it, what did you replace it with?
10. How did it feel when you exchanged it or released the coat?
11. How does this relate to protection in your present life?
12. What do you feel you need to protect yourself from at present?

CREATIVE SELF

"This world is but a canvas to our imagination" ~ Henry David Thoreau

You are walking on an earthen path with beautiful trees on each side of you. You feel a sense of peace as you walk the path among the graceful trees, listening to the birds sing . . . smelling the fresh scent of green. You walk down the path as it weaves itself to an opening, where you see a beautiful meadow. You continue walking, relaxed and energized.

Entering the meadow you see the tall grass swaying, and flowers of vivid colors blow gently in the breeze as far as you can see. You smell the clean, fresh earth and hear the tall grass swishing in the breeze as you walk. The air brushes against your face. Up above, white clouds move slowly through the bluest sky you've ever seen. Everything feels alive. You hear chimes ringing and beautiful music in the distance. Feel the magic around you in this beautiful place. You are enlivened by the air you breathe . . . life flowing through you, at one with all.

You continue on the pathway to a small pond ahead. The breeze gently ripples the water, and it shimmers, reflecting the sun. You walk over to the pond and bend down next to the water. As you look down into the water, your own reflection catches your attention.

Suddenly, your reflection comes alive in the water. Your reflection smiles at you and says "I am your Creative Self." Your reflection says, "I am limitless in ideas and creative expression. There is no beginning or end; creation flows through me as you allow. Will you allow me to flow through you?"

Your Creative Self becomes animate and stands in front of you on the shore.

(Note: Please pause after each question to allow the participant to visualize and process.)

1. With great love, your Creative Self hands you a gift. Look closely at it, feel it, and touch it. What is the gift?
2. How can you use this gift in your life?
3. And now, you give your Creative Self a gift. What is the gift you give?
4. And what does this gift mean to you?

Now, your Creative Self reminds you that they are a very important part of you. They embrace you. You enjoy the feeling of the energy moving between you. You now feel their essence enter you and integrate into you. You feel the alive, abundant, and creative energy flowing throughout your entire body. You look out at the vibrant meadow and give thanks, knowing that upon your return to this room, you *are* creative energy flowing outward, creating this world. Enjoy the sensation and this feeling of flow.

And now, beginning to return . . . remembering everything you saw and experienced clearly . . . as I begin to count up from one to five . . . Counting up one . . . and two . . . feeling more alert . . . relaxed and refreshed from this creative journey within . . . Up three and four . . . bringing your gifts to life . . . as life brings its gift to you . . . from the outside in and the inside out . . . Beginning to stretch your fingers and toes . . . and opening your eyes on the count to five, feeling alive, vital, and inspired.

CONNECT TO CREATIVITY

PURPOSE: *CREATIVITY*

SUMMARY: Connect with your creativity and the gifts you have to share with the world. Exchange gifts and receive a message from your Creative Self.

MY EXPERIENCE: I enjoy utilizing this imagery with clients in recovery so they can verbally reconnect with their creativity. It is common to hear people say that they have lost their creativity or are not as creative when they are not using. Dialoguing can be the beginning of forward movement. You can also have participant(s) journal or do artwork or collage after imagery.

EXAMPLE: Kathryn has felt out of touch with her creativity and enjoyed seeing her Creative Self. Her Creative Self was at first hazy and unclear. Her Creative Self gave her a beautiful painting of a heart, and in return, Kathryn gave her paints and paint brushes. She was surprised that after giving her Creative Self the paint brushes, she became clear and vivid. Her Creative Self said, "Please let me paint; we'll both be happier."

CREATIVE SELF: INSIGHT PAGE QUESTIONS

1. How did your Creative Self present itself to you?
2. What was your impression of your Creative Self?
3. Was there anything that stood out?
4. What gift did your Creative Self give you?
5. How can you use and share this gift with others?
6. What was the gift you gave in return?
7. What message did your Creative Self give you?
8. What does this mean to you?
9. How can you use it in relation to your creativity?
10. What does the use of your creativity give to you and to those around you?

CRYING CHILD

"Our sorrows and wounds are healed only when we touch them with compassion." ~ Buddha

Allowing yourself to get very comfortable now . . . Closing your eyes as you're ready . . . Letting all your muscles open up . . . expand . . . and relax. Noticing that there is a light of the most beautiful color surrounding your entire body. You take in a healing breath, as you inhale peace and calm from this light. Feeling and seeing it all around you. Inhaling peace, exhaling calm. Inhaling calm, exhaling peace. Absorbing the peace and calm as you breathe. Absorbing the healing properties as it moves through your mind . . . down through your heart . . . brightening and glowing . . . down through your arms . . . into your hands . . . Through your stomach . . . shimmering and sparkling . . . through your abdomen and into your legs . . . into the bottom of your feet . . . Filled with peace and calm . . . And now going softly, safely . . . into the imagination . . .

Imagine that you, as a child, are in your childhood room crying. Your father walks in the door.

(Note: Please pause at each step to allow the participant to visualize and process.)

1. How does he react to your crying?
2. And how does that feel?

Now let that scene fade . . . Again, you are crying in that room, and your mother walks in the door.

3. How does *she* react to your crying?
4. And how does that feel?
5. Now tell your father how his reactions have affected you as an adult.
6. Tell him how you use that experience in a positive way in your adult life.
7. Now tell your mother how her reactions have affected you as an adult.
8. And how you use that in a positive way in your adult life.

And now, imagine that you, as the adult you are now with all your gained wisdom and experience, step into that room.

9. How do you feel as you see that child crying?
10. Comfort the child now in whatever way you choose. Say whatever you need to say to them.
11. Be aware of how your child-self responds to your support.
12. Let them know that *you* are taking care of them now and want the very best for them.

And now, beginning to return to room awareness, aware of the surface below you . . . as you prepare to come back. Hearing sounds in and outside the room . . . and the sound of my voice . . . Becoming aware of your breathing, relaxed and regular . . . Feeling light and more alert. Taking in a breath of energizing oxygen, and you bring yourself back to room awareness, refreshed and rejuvenated, enlightened and at peace . . . As you open your eyes now . . . to the light of the room . . .

REPARENT INNER CHILD

PURPOSE: *INNER CHILD*

CAVEAT: If you are working with a participant with trauma, determine whether this imagery is appropriate for the participant.

SUMMARY: As an adult, the participant visits their crying inner child and witnesses their father's and mother's respective reactions to crying. Their adult-self comforts their child-self. Adult-self tells their parents how their reactions affected them in their adult life and how they are using this in the positive now.

MY EXPERIENCE: This imagery often brings tears and compassion to clients for their inner child. Within the imagery, they have the opportunity to feel their inner child's vulnerability and feel their desire to reparent and love them now.

EXAMPLE: Within the imagery, Hunter watches his father respond to his crying by yelling, "I'll give you something to cry about!" and raising a fist to him. He feels sorry for the child, comforts him, and feels his father's frustration and inability to deal with emotions. His mother reacts by placing her arms around him and saying, "It'll be okay, you're fine." He tells his child-self that he loves him and that he's taking care of him now.

CRYING CHILD: INSIGHT PAGE QUESTIONS

1. Approximately how old was your child-self? What was happening at that time in your life?
2. How did you feel as your child-self cried?
3. How did your father react to your crying? How do you feel about that?
4. And how has that affected your life?
5. How do you use it positively in your life at present?
6. How did your mother react to your crying? How do you feel about that?
7. And how has that affected your life?
8. How do you use it positively in your life at present?
9. How did it feel when you, as the adult, comforted that crying child?
10. How did your child-self respond to your support?
11. What did you tell the child?
12. How can you use this information in your present life?

CUBE

"Our whole life is solving puzzles." ~ Erno Rubik

Getting settled into the surface you're on now . . . closing your eyes. Taking in a long, deep healing breath, inhaling from your stomach up into your chest . . . and releasing it as you let go of all of the day's thoughts and concerns . . . Drifting down into a soothing state of serenity . . . Taking in another deep breath . . . and exhaling anything unlike peace and serenity . . . Feeling centered, soothed, and content . . . Breathing in one more deep breath . . . into the stomach . . . up into the chest . . . and releasing it . . . as you rest into the stillness . . . your body and mind drifting . . . into relaxation . . . with all senses soothed . . . drifting deeper . . . into the imagination . . .

And now you see that you're under the most perfect blue sky, walking on a path in an open space of land and sky . . . And ahead, you see a cube. You are curious . . . and begin walking toward the cube.

(Note: Please pause between each question to allow participant to visualize and process.)

1. What size is the cube? How is it placed on the landscape?
2. What color is it?
3. And what is it made of?
4. You can walk around it now to see all sides of it and even touch it. How does the texture of the cube feel?
5. As you walk completely around it, you notice that there is a ladder near the cube. What is the ladder made of?
6. You decide to climb the ladder. Begin stepping up each rung of the ladder to the top. Notice how it feels as you use it to get to the top.
7. And now, on top of the cube, how do you feel?
8. You can choose to do anything you like there at the top of the cube.
9. Look out and notice what you see in the distance.

And now, you decide to go back down the ladder. Climb down, one rung at a time. As you touch your feet on the ground and turn around, you see a horse coming toward you.

10. What does this horse look like?
11. What is its size and color?
12. How do you feel about it?
13. How close do you choose to get to it?
14. And how does the horse respond to you?

Interact with the horse in any way you choose. And now, you look up to the sky and notice there is a storm coming. What do you do?

And now, beginning to return to room consciousness . . . Becoming more aware of your breath. Hearing my words and the sounds in and outside . . . Beginning to stretch your arms and legs. Taking in a refreshing breath, feeling more alert. Remembering everything you saw and experienced clearly. Moving your fingers and toes . . . Feeling rejuvenated and revitalized . . . Counting up one . . . and two . . . up three and four . . . And now . . . gently opening your eyes on the count of five . . . Refreshed, rejuvenated, and ready for the rest of the day.

SELF, SUPPORT SYSTEM, LOVE, CHALLENGES

PURPOSE: *SELF-DISCOVERY*

SUMMARY: The participant can receive information regarding their beliefs about self, support, activity, love, trust, and challenges as they see and describe a cube (self), ladder (support), horse (love/trust), and storm (challenges). As with all other imageries, do not tell the participant(s) what the cube represents prior to imagery. See the USD for more information (color, etc.). *Note: This imagery was modified from the book* The Cube *(see Resources).*

MY EXPERIENCE: Clients have fun and gain self-awareness with this imagery. It is great for group work, as an icebreaker, and for journaling. It takes longer than most, so if working with more than five people, give yourself more than an hour.

EXAMPLE: David sees a cube (self) of transparent glass. He thinks it's "cool" but is concerned when he climbs the ladder (support) to the top and sees a few cracks. As he runs his hand over the cracks, they are repaired, and he is amazed. He climbs down the ladder to see a beautiful, but wild brown horse (love/trust) that is rearing up and neighing. He is drawn to it and frightened at the same time. When the storm (challenge) comes, David looks to the horse, which allows him to jump on its back. They ride away from the storm. David reviews the imagery's meaning. He thinks that he's being more transparent (glass). He is working on healing himself (cracks repairing when he pays attention). He says that he has a good support system (sturdy ladder). He laughs about the wild horse as he says he is drawn to dramatic relationships. He explains that he's still working on setting healthy boundaries and not expecting a relationship to save him during challenges.

CUBE: INSIGHT PAGE QUESTIONS

Cube (self and one's view of self)
1. Describe your cube. What size was it? What color? What was it made of?
2. What was the texture? And how did it feel if you touched it?
3. What did you think of the cube? What did you like and dislike about it?

Ladder (support system, self/others)
4. What was the ladder made of? What do you think of this material?
5. Was it leaning against the cube, or was it attached?
6. Did it feel stable as you climbed up?

Top of the Cube (activity level: sitting/standing/lying down)
7. What did you do at the top of the cube? And how did you feel?

Horse (love/trust)
8. Describe the horse. What size was it? What color? What were the horse's qualities?
9. How close did you get to the horse? How did you interact?
10. How did you feel about the horse? And how did it feel about you?

Storm (challenges)
11. Describe the storm; how you felt about it, and what you decided to do.

DIRECTOR

"You only have control over three things in your life—the thoughts you think, the images you visualize, and the actions you take." ~ Jack Canfield

Close your eyes as you relax into the surface you're on and feel how it supports you completely. As I count from five down to one, becoming more relaxed with each breath you take in ... and release ... Counting five and four ... Feeling peace flowing through every cell in your body ... from your head down through your neck, into your shoulders, arms, and hands ... Deeper relaxed, three and two ... knowing that your life is in your hands. Down through your chest, stomach, and back, down through your legs, and way down to one, into your ankles and into your feet. Feeling so relaxed ...

You have completed writing the script of your life to the present time, and you're now beginning to realize that you are sitting in the director's chair ... that you are the director of your own life.

After years, it felt as though you were practicing life in a sense—pretending to live it, but not fully. As if awakening from a dream, you've realized how important your life is and how important you are. Writing about your life can be enlightening and powerful. You understand that you are the writer of your life, continually imagining it, directing it, and editing it. Being the director, you have the authority to choose which actors play a part. You choose who participates in your life story. You have the choice to let go of bad actors and to edit out those things that don't improve your life script. You have the final say.

You have been making progress. You're concentrating more on you, the most important person in your life. You are surrounding yourself with supportive people who want the best for you and your life's vision.

You have become aware that there is an actor in your life script that you haven't communicated with honestly. Allow this person to appear in your mind now, just allowing it to be who it is. You decide that you can talk with this person in the rehearsal room of your mind. You realize that in your position as writer and director of your own life that you have complete authority, and even the responsibility, to talk directly with them in order to have a better relationship and understanding of one another. Imagine that you sit in your director's chair right now. And this person comes to talk with you at your request. They sit down in a chair directly across from you.

1. Tell them that it's important for you to be direct and honest with them.
2. And now, say what you need to say, with kindness and clarity, as the director of your life. *(Note: Give ample time for participant to experience.)*
3. How do you feel after speaking your truth?

Know that in the reality of your life, you have the authority to take action on this.

And now, beginning to return ... remembering everything you saw and experienced ... Counting up from one to five ... Counting up one ... and two ... feeling more alert ... relaxed and refreshed, up three and four ... from the outside in and the inside out ... Beginning to stretch your fingers and toes ... and opening your eyes on the count to five, feeling lighter, in control, directing your life ... Counting five ... Opening your eyes ... Revitalized.

HONEST COMMUNICATION IN RELATIONSHIP

PURPOSE: *RELATIONSHIPS*

SUMMARY: The participant sits in the director's chair, realizing that they are the writer, editor, and director of their own life. They become aware that they have the ability, and in fact, the responsibility, to be honest and clear in their communication. They choose to speak to a person whom they feel they have not been openly honest with.

MY EXPERIENCE: This imagery can be empowering and/or uncomfortable for the participants as they are given control of a relationship or situation to practice. I have also had clients comment that this imagery reminded them that they do have more control than they previously thought.

EXAMPLE: Diane says she has never thought of herself as the director of her own life, and she liked the concept. She chose to communicate with her grandmother in the imagery, whom she said can be extremely negative at times. Diane imagined herself telling her grandmother that she often feels depressed after talking with her and would prefer to talk about more positive things in the future. Diane said it felt good practicing telling her the truth and that she plans to write down notes to prepare herself for a call to her grandmother.

DIRECTOR: INSIGHT PAGE QUESTIONS

1. How did it feel to think of yourself as the Director of Your Life?
2. Who was the person in your life that you need to communicate with and for what reason?
3. How did it feel speaking to the person in the rehearsal room of your mind?
4. How did you feel when you finished speaking the truth?
5. How can you use this information to take action on things you want to edit or change in your life story?

FOREST OF FORGIVENESS

"It's one of the greatest gifts you can give yourself, to forgive. Forgive everybody." ~ Maya Angelou

Close your eyes and take in a deep relaxation breath, into your stomach . . . and up into your chest, and release it . . . as you let go of all the day's thoughts and concerns . . . anything that isn't right here and right now . . . Releasing . . . allowing all the muscles in your body to relax deeply . . . Letting go of sounds in and outside . . . Going within and imagining yourself in the most beautiful forest . . . Smelling the earth . . .

You now stand in an opening under a canopy of towering redwood trees. Breathe in the musky-clean fragrance of the rich brown earth beneath you. Feeling grounded and supported, you look at the sacred cathedral of ancient trees above you. Cool mists of fog slowly flow through the tall green branches reaching outward above you. Translucent ferns and feathered moss fill the soft green floor of the forest. A waft of fog-dampened air refreshes you, while the cleansing scent of pine soothes your senses.

As you walk the path toward the lofty trees climbing into the sky, you see a person on the path ahead who might have hurt or betrayed you who needs forgiveness.

(Note: Please pause after each question to give the participant time to visualize and process.)

    1. Who is this person?

There they stand in silence in this gentle, nourishing forest. The fog above them begins to disperse and a shaft of light shines down through the trees. You walk toward the warmth of the light glowing all around this person. As you get closer, you see the light of their soul shining in their eyes.

Suddenly, you see them become a child, innocent and curious. You know they are in need of something they didn't receive.

    2. What is it that they needed as a child that they did not get?

You remind yourself that they are only human. And their humanness softens your soul. As you approach them, you are connected with the light above. The warmth of the higher energy fills the space connecting you. You feel the power and the opportunity of forgiveness. You feel a shift in energy as you align with the flow of light, reminding you to let go, so the two of you may walk your paths ahead in peace, whether you share the path or not.

This person stands in front of you now, at their present age. Take this time to forgive this person in any way you choose, with words, actions, feelings. (ample pause)

    3. How do they respond?
    4. Tell them something that you admire and appreciate about them.
    5. And now they, in turn, tell you what they admire and appreciate about you.
    6. Tell them what you have learned from your journey together.
    7. Tell them how you might best move forward in friendship, love, or work, and allow them to respond.

Say goodbye in whatever way you choose now. Feel the bright, glowing light of love and forgiveness flow through you. Look up and around this beautiful cathedral of trees, bringing back remembrances of all that is good. Counting up one and two . . . Knowing you are able and capable of change, three and four . . . Giving yourself and others the gift of forgiveness . . . Becoming aware of the room . . . Feeling the lightness, openness, and awareness. And counting five, opening your eyes to the light of the room.

FORGIVE ANOTHER OR YOURSELF

PURPOSE: *FORGIVENESS*

SUMMARY: Forgive yourself or another. See the person as a child and understand what they did not receive. Tell this person what you admire about them and what you have learned from them in your time together.

MY EXPERIENCE: The forgiveness given is often self-forgiveness. Clients sometimes cry during this imagery and see unexpected people to forgive.

EXAMPLE: Lucy sees her father in the forest. Her father appears as a child, looking lonely and scared. Lucy knows that her father needed love that he didn't receive. Lucy tells her father that she is grateful that he didn't abandon her as his father did, and she expresses her love to him. Lucy verbally forgives her father for not being the person she wanted him to be and hugs him. She suggests that they continue to try to understand one another, even though they are very different people.

ADAPTATION: You can adapt this imagery for self-forgiveness or forgiveness of a chosen person (pre-chosen by the participant).

FOREST OF FORGIVENESS: INSIGHT PAGE QUESTIONS

1. Who appeared in the forest that had hurt or betrayed you and needed forgiveness?
2. How did they appear as you approached them, and how did you feel?
3. How did you feel as you looked at them as a child? What did they need as that child?
4. What did you tell them that you admire and appreciate about them? How did they respond?
5. What did they tell you that they admire and appreciate about you? How did you respond?
6. What did you tell them you learned from them?
7. In what way did you forgive them?
8. What did you tell them was needed to move forward in the best way?
9. How did you feel after the forgiveness (and apology if one was given)?
10. How can you use this to better your life and the other person's?

FUTURE SELF

"Do something today that your future self will thank you for." ~ Unknown

And now, you find that you are on the most beautiful beach . . . The air is the perfect temperature. You watch the sparkling waves come in to the shore, the white foam disappearing into the wet sand . . . reflecting the sun . . . The sun shimmers on the water . . . You breathe in the perfect ocean air . . . with the slight scent of salt . . . So healing and refreshing . . . Relaxing deeper as I count from five down to one . . . Feeling more and more relaxed with each word I say . . . Down to four . . . More relaxed with each breath you take and release . . . You hear the booming sound of the waves coming in to the shore . . . And then . . . soothing silence . . . The sound of a seagull in the distance . . . Feeling more relaxed, down to . . . three . . . so at peace . . . Counting two . . . and down to one, so serene.

You are strolling along the shore, feeling the damp sand under your feet as you walk. Up ahead, you see your future self walking toward you. The future you looks happy, healthy, confident, with a wide smile on their face. Getting closer, you notice the confidence and joy they radiate. You can feel the love they have for you and see it in their eyes. They want only the very best for you and are grateful that you led them to health and happiness.

Your future self puts their arms around you and gives you a warm and comforting hug. You can feel their heartbeat, their essence, and their love.

(Note: Please pause after each question to allow the participant to visualize and process.)

1. Your future self whispers into your ear and tells you. What actions you took to become so healthy and confidenct.
2. They give you a gift you need for your present and future health.
3. You now give them a gift of gratitude for your health.
4. Thank them for their gift, their love, and their positive *actions*.

Now you place your arms around them to connect again. And as you do, you feel their energy, intention, and vitality move into your body as brilliant light . . . moving into your heart, up through your mind, down your arms, and into your hands. Down through the center of you, filled with all intelligence and information needed to live your healthiest life. Down through your legs, moving you forward in healthy beliefs, thoughts, and actions.

And now, beginning to return to room awareness, aware of the surface under you . . . Counting up one . . . and two . . . as you prepare to come back. Hearing sounds in and outside the room . . . the sound of my voice . . . Becoming aware of your breathing . . . Counting up three . . . Feeling light and alert. Taking in a breath of energizing oxygen, coming back, refreshed and rejuvenated . . . Counting four . . . Revitalized and renewed . . . And as I count to five . . . opening your eyes . . . to the light of the room . . .

EXPERIENCE YOURSELF, AS YOU WISH TO BE

PURPOSE: *MOTIVATION*

SUMMARY: Receive guidance from your future self and exchange gifts needed for the future.

MY EXPERIENCE: Inspires people in transition and encourages goal setting through experiencing success.

EXAMPLE: Andre saw himself two years into the future. He looked healthy, strong, and happy, with his eyes shining brightly. His future self told him, "Keep doing what you're doing; you'll get here. Life is good!" What stood out to Andre was his future self's genuine smile and the feeling of love when he hugged him. He said, "It felt good to feel so proud of myself."

ADAPTATION: This imagery can be adapted to any attribute wanted in the future.

FUTURE SELF: INSIGHT PAGE QUESTIONS

1. Describe seeing your future self approach you.
2. How did your future self look? And how did it feel to see them?
3. What qualities did your future self have?
4. What small details did you notice?
5. How did it feel when they embraced you?
6. What information did your future self give you?
7. What gift did your future self give you?
8. What gift of gratitude did you give them?
9. What actions can you take toward living a happier, healthier life?

GARDEN OF GRATITUDE

"Gratitude unlocks the fullness of life. It turns what we have into enough, and more.
It turns denial into acceptance, chaos into order, confusion into clarity.
It can turn a meal into a feast, a house into a home, a stranger into a friend." ~ Melody Beattie

Settling into the surface you're on . . . Letting your body completely relax into gravity. Closing your eyes as you take in a deep relaxation breath . . . allowing all of your muscles to expand and let go . . . taking another relaxation breath and releasing it. Giving yourself complete permission to relax and rest into the stillness of the moment . . . into your center, in the here and now. Gently breathing in and out, out and in, as your breathing becomes slower . . . shifting attention inward, into the center of calm and contentment within you. Your mind and body at peace, as you move deeper into that center to allow yourself to wonder and wander . . . As you drift down to observe and absorb the quiet . . . in the center . . . of the soothing . . . silence . . . within . . .

Sometimes we forget to remember the good we have and remember only what we don't have. It can be distracting, and it's not surprising, because we're taught to want . . . and that's okay. It's just a matter of focus, of turning it around . . . Focusing on the good, planting seeds of gratitude, and nourishing the good that is already there. And now . . .

You see yourself planting a garden of gratitude. You're placing seeds into small open circles in the dark fertile soil of your garden. You're gently filling in the dirt over them and nourishing them with water. Smelling that clean, fresh scent of earth. And like the seeds of gratitude, we can't always see what's growing underneath . . . until the seeds send roots through the dark fertile soil, growing stronger, reaching up through the earth, toward the sun, into beauty and grace. And now, time has passed, and the seeds have borne flowers in full bloom.

(Note: Please pause after each question to give participant time to visualize and process.)

1. You stand looking at these beautiful flowers in your garden of gratitude.
2. Look closely at one of them. What type of flower is it?
3. Touch the flower and feel its texture . . . enjoy its shape and color.
4. If it has a fragrance, breathe in that scent and enjoy it.

As you look at the beautiful flower, you imagine a person whom you are grateful for and to.

5. Imagine that they stand with you now, smiling, near your beautiful garden.
6. Tell them that you are grateful to have them in your life.
7. Tell them what they have brought to you . . . and how it makes you feel.
8. Embrace them, and thank them in whatever way feels comfortable.
9. Say whatever else you'd like to say to them. And say goodbye for now.

It feels good *not* think of what we *don't* want . . . to love what we *do have*, to create beauty *right here* where we are. Sharing gestures of gratitude: a call of words . . . with actions . . . and service . . . written notes, a homemade card, a drawing. Gratitude seeds through words and deeds, to nurture and grow through sun or snow . . .

And now, feeling more aware as you prepare to come back to room consciousness . . . Hearing my words and the sounds in and outside of the room. Beginning to stretch your arms and legs and take in a refreshing breath of air, oxygenating your body. Feeling light, relaxed into the present of the moment . . . Focused and aware . . . Feeling relaxed and renewed from this journey within. Remembering everything you saw and experienced . . . Becoming more alert as you stretch your body and bring yourself back to room awareness by opening your eyes to the light of the room . . . Refreshed and rejuvenated.

EXPRESSING GRATITUDE

PURPOSE: *ACCEPTANCE, GRATITUDE*

SUMMARY: Plant a metaphoric garden and express gratitude to a person you are thankful for. *Note: The flower is the symbol within the imagery. After asking the Insight questions, you can look the flower up in the Universal Symbol Dictionary for other qualities.*

MY EXPERIENCE: This imagery is a good rehearsal for expressing gratitude to someone whom the participant would like to thank, especially if there is some embarrassment or guilt attached to it.

EXAMPLE: Laura plants yellow roses in her garden and loves their scent and beauty. She sees her mother in the imagery. She feels so grateful for the sacrifices her mother made to benefit her and her sisters. She said it felt great to express her gratitude because she hasn't done that enough in the past.

GARDEN OF GRATITUDE: INSIGHT PAGE QUESTIONS

1. What flower did you see in your garden of gratitude?
2. Does this flower have any special meaning to you? What does it bring to mind?
3. Who was the person you feel grateful for?
4. What did you thank them for?
5. What was their reaction?
6. And how does that make you feel?

GUIDE

"We have a better guide in ourselves,
if we would attend it, than any person can be."~ Jane Austen

Gently closing your eyes . . . getting into a comfortable position . . . as comfortable as you need to be. Taking in a deep breath and letting it go, along with anything that isn't right here and right now. Allowing the day to take care of itself for a while, or even longer. Taking in another breath and releasing it. Giving yourself complete permission to take this time to imagine yourself drifting down a slow and lazy river in a small and comfy boat. Slowly, safely flowing under a canopy of trees. Watching the bright green leaves shimmer under the sun and light dance off the slow-moving water. The river of relaxation flows within you and under you as you drift gently, calmly with the river. Flowing onward, slowing down, into a beautiful lake, where you can float and relax with all the time in the world. Smelling the fresh, cleansing fragrance of the water and the healing scent of pine, hearing the sound of the water lapping on the shore in that timeless way . . . Nothing to do . . . nowhere to be. Simply slowing down . . . safe . . . secure . . . and serene . . .

And now, you're standing on the shore beside the quiet lake.

(Note: Please pause after each question to allow the participant time to visualize and process.)

Feeling very safe in this beautiful place, invite an unconditionally loving guide to be with you . . . one who is wise and kind and knows you better than you know yourself. And now your guide stands in front of you. Get a very clear picture of your guide and greet them in any way you choose.

1. Notice your guide's qualities . . . and how you feel around this being.
2. Ask your guide what name they would like to be called.
3. Ask them if they will be available to you in times of need. Ask them anything you feel is important at present . . .
4. Thank them for their information, and say goodbye in any way you choose, knowing you can always connect with them again when needed.

And now, feeling the surface under you. Hearing the sounds around you . . . Feeling comfortable, content. Remembering everything you saw and experienced . . . Relaxed, calm, and centered. Beginning to stretch your fingers and toes, counting up one and two . . . feeling peaceful and focused as you return to room awareness . . . More aware and alert, three and four . . . And beginning to open your eyes as I say . . . the number . . . five . . . And . . . opening your eyes . . . to the light of the room . . . refreshed, rejuvenated, and ready for the rest of the day.

MEET A WISE, SUPPORTIVE GUIDE

PURPOSE: *SELF-DISCOVERY*

SUMMARY: Meet a supportive and loving guide who has answers for you, whom you can call upon when needed.

MY EXPERIENCE: This simple imagery can be powerful and poignant as it connects people with their faith and spirituality. I have seen many people shed joyful tears when they connect with their guides. Their guide can be a staunch supporter, a comfort, an inner-therapist, and an inspiration.

EXAMPLE: Mateo visualized Quan Yin as his guide, and he said he could feel the compassion and love that she had for him. Quan Yin told Mateo, "Have compassion for yourself. Love yourself as I do." Mateo said that when he asked Quan Yin if she would be available when he needed her, she answered, "I am always with you. Just ask and I'll appear."

GUIDE: INSIGHT PAGE QUESTIONS

1. Describe your guide.
2. What were the qualities of your guide?
3. What was your guide's name?
4. How did your guide react to giving you support during times of need?
5. What information did your guide give you regarding your question?
6. How did you say goodbye?

HALL OF FALSE BELIEFS

"Work on being in love with the person in the mirror
who has been through so much but is still standing." ~ Anonymous

And now, beginning to relax as I count from five down to one . . . Feeling more and more relaxed with each word I say . . . And even the spaces between my words . . . Down to four . . . more and more relaxed with each descending number . . . Each breath you take and release . . . Each beat of your heart . . . Even more relaxed to three . . . Deeper relaxed . . . Calming . . . quieting . . . Counting two . . . and down to one. Very safe and so relaxed . . .

You, with all your adult experience, knowledge, and wisdom, find yourself in front of a large building called the Hall of False Beliefs. You are curious about this building.

You begin walking up the steps to the entrance and see your own name up above the door with the words *False Beliefs* below it. You open the door and begin walking down the hall. You notice that on each side of the hallway are doors with past experiences that created false beliefs. You walk until you come to a door that has a specific label or belief that has had the most effect on you. Notice what this false label is.

Knowing you are now safe enough to address it in your imagination, step inside the room and watch this past experience like a movie. You have a remote control in your hand, so you have the power to play the movie forward, or pause it where you choose. Press *play* when you're ready and allow yourself to watch an earlier version of you within that experience. (ample pause)

(Note: Please pause after each step to allow the participant time to visualize and process.)

1. When that younger you feels the emotional response to this false belief, pause the action, and step over to speak to them from your present viewpoint.
2. Get their attention and greet them in whatever way you choose.
3. Now, tell your younger self that they were given *erroneous* information.
4. Place your arms around that younger self and comfort them.
5. You know how they feel better than anyone else.
6. Thank them for the strength it took to get through this earlier time.
7. Tell them that this false label is not the truth of who they are.
8. Tell them the good of who they really are. *(ample pause)*
9. And now, give them a new, positive label that is more appropriate.
10. Take their hand, look at them, and restate their new, positive label, saying, "You are . . ." How do they respond?
11. Now, walk out of the hall with your younger self. How do they feel?
12. Embrace them again, feeling the reality of this new, positive label. Allow them, with their new self-regard—like light—to integrate into you: mind, body, and spirit.

And now, beginning to return . . . Remembering everything you saw and experienced clearly . . . As I begin to count up from one to five . . . Counting up one . . . and two . . . Feeling more alert . . . Relaxed and refreshed from this journey within . . . Up three and four . . . Beginning to stretch your fingers and toes . . . Feeling revitalized and renewed . . . And opening your eyes on the count of five, ready for the rest of the day.

REFRAME AND RENAME A FALSE BELIEF

PURPOSE: *RELEASE, SELF-LOVE*

SUMMARY: Identify a false belief/label, have a dialogue with your former self, reframe, and rename the false label or belief from the past.

MY EXPERIENCE: Everyone has a false belief or label from the past that they can benefit from changing. This imagery offers the participant a way to reframe and release a false belief to whatever degree possible at this time. The new, positive label can be reinforced with a writing activity, affirmations, or positive suggestions.

EXAMPLE: Al is almost sixty years old. He sees a door labeled *Not Good Enough* and walks in to see his father, who never gave him a compliment or told him that he loved him. Al tells his younger self, "You *are* good enough; you're far better than good enough! Your father didn't really know you." Al gives himself a new label: *Great*. His child-self smiles at his adult-self and feels good as they leave the Hall of False Beliefs.

HALL OF FALSE BELIEFS: INSIGHT PAGE QUESTIONS

1. How did you feel walking into the Hall of False Beliefs?
2. Describe the hall. Approximately how many doors were there?
3. What was the belief/label on the door you chose to go in?
4. What happened in the room? What situation created the false belief?
5. What did you tell your former self about this false belief, and how did your former self respond?
6. What was the new belief or positive label you chose for yourself?
7. As you walked out of the door of the Hall of False Beliefs with your previous self and new positive label/belief, how did you feel?
8. How do you feel as you say this new positive belief to yourself: "I am . . ."?
9. How can you use this in your present life?

HEALING TEMPLE

"First, every day I would put all my conscious attention on this intelligence within me and give it a plan, a template, a vision with very specific orders, and then I would surrender my healing to this greater mind that has unlimited power, to do the healing for me." ~ Joe Dispenza

Gently closing your eyes . . . Taking in a cleansing breath and releasing it. Allowing yourself to slow down into silence . . . As you see and feel the most peaceful, violet light shining around the crown of your head . . . Filled with soothing serenity . . . Breathe it in. Feel it permeate your head, as it turns into the most beautiful purple light . . . as all the tiny muscles around your eyes and mouth go smooth and relaxed . . . The purple light moves down into your neck, becoming a soothing, calming blue. Breathe it into your throat, as all muscles in your neck relax . . . Your shoulders relax into gravity, as the light moves down into your chest . . . as the light becomes a harmonious, healing green, flowing through your heart and lungs and back . . . through your arms . . . into your hands. Healing green flows down toward your center, becoming the brightest, happiest yellow. Into your abdomen . . . and through the small of your back, becoming a bright citrus orange. Flowing through your hips and buttocks, glowing with life-giving red. Deeper relaxed, down through your thighs, your knees, and your legs . . . becoming a brilliant scarlet. Through all muscles, tendons, and bone . . . healing, revitalizing, down through your ankles into your feet . . . Becoming the most healing earthy brown . . . Relaxed . . . Grounded . . . Filled with light . . . healing . . . transformation . . .

And now you come upon the most beautiful healing temple, created especially for you as your body temple knows exactly what you need in the here and now. You see healing pools, where water of one specific color flows over a wall of healing words into the healing pool you can float in. The air is magical—the most perfect temperature. Healing plants and trees surround the temple, and you breathe in the most fragrant healing scents. You hear tranquil music coming from every direction, created just for you. Feeling the vibrations of the music attuning to your body, each cell resonating in harmony . . .

You get into the healing pool with the beautiful water of the perfect temperature. You can swim, float, or sit under the healing words as the water flows down into the pool you sit in.

(Note: Please pause after each question to allow the practitioner to visualize and process.)

1. How does the water feel? What color is the water?
2. What word or phrase do you see on the healing wall?
3. You notice a symbol carved into the wall that means something to you and your health.

The magical healing water flowing through the pool removes anything from your body that is no longer needed as it moves down through a gentle drain at the bottom of the pool. A sparkling, healing light within you goes to the place in your body that needs it most. See this brilliant light of health and healing shimmer and sparkle in your cells down to the bones, to the DNA, absorbing this light, rebuilding as the body does naturally, life renewing life. As you relax in the water, so soothed and serene, every cell in your body enlightened with strength, comfort, and vitality.

Now bringing your healthy self back into the present. Remembering everything you saw and experienced . . . Breathing in fresh oxygen, vital and energizing . . . Beginning to move your fingers and toes . . . Stretching as you need . . . Feeling radiant. Embodying health and vitality. Glowing from the inside out and the outside in . . . To return to room awareness . . . Relaxed, rejuvenated, revitalized . . . As you open your eyes.

VISIT A HEALING TEMPLE

PURPOSE: *HEALTH, WELLNESS*

SUMMARY: Visit a healing temple. Bathe in the healing water. Receive a message regarding health from the words/phrases and a symbol on the healing wall. Experience health and wellbeing.

MY EXPERIENCE: This is a soothing imagery for clients feeling anxiety or physical discomfort. If you'd like to give a deeper relaxation experience, you can repeat the healing portion of the imagery starting at entering the pool and (if working with an individual) adding their own peaceful place if you choose. (Ask prior to imagery). This imagery is also beneficial as *remembered wellness* for an immune boost.

EXAMPLE: Tracy imagines herself in turquoise water, which she says represents tranquility. She sees a phrase on the healing wall that reads, "To thine own self be true." She believes this means that she needs to focus her attention on her own health now instead of using her energy on other life distractions that take her time.

HEALING TEMPLE: INSIGHT PAGE QUESTIONS

1. Describe the healing temple.
2. What color was the water in the healing pool?
3. What does this color represent to you?
4. What were the healing words or the phrases on the wall that the water poured over?
5. How do these words relate to your healing and health?
6. If you saw a symbol on the healing wall, what was it and do you know what it means?
7. What did the healing water take from your body that it no longer needs?
8. How can you use this information to feel your best?

HEALTHY SELF

"Keeping your body healthy is an expression of gratitude to the whole cosmos—
the trees, the clouds, everything." ~ Thich Nhat Hanh

It is the most beautiful day on the beach: the perfect temperature and time of day. You look toward the sea and breathe in the fresh salt air. The sky is blue and cloudless. Your toes are in the warm, soft sand as a breeze moves over your body. You watch as the sun shimmers and dances off the clean, clear blue expanse of water. You watch the waves roll into shore and hear that soft roar, and then . . . the soothing silence. The waves come in and out, in and out, in that timeless rhythm of life. White foam disappears into the wet sand as it reflects the light of the sun. You feel the slight mist of the ocean as you relax even deeper. The palm trees rustle in the breeze, and you hear the sound of people talking in the distance, but it doesn't matter. You are so completely relaxed . . .

You decide to take a walk along the beach. You walk the shore alone, appreciating the openness and the soothing sounds, scents, and sights of the sea. As you continue to walk, peaceful and relaxed, you see your healthy self walking toward you. This is you, at your ultimate health. Luminous, happy, strong, and vital. Your healthy self—radiant, with a vibrant smile—comes close to greet you.

(Note: Please pause after each question to allow the participant time to visualize and process.)

1. Enjoy this time with your healthy self. Look at your healthy self and notice details: Their clothing. Their qualities and attitude. The health and vitality of their body.
2. Observe their physicality.
3. Feel their essence.
4. Ask your healthy self, "How have I become you?" and listen to their answer.
5. Thank your healthy self for their information and ask anything else you need to know.

Now, your healthy self thanks you and tells you that they are already there within you. They put their arms around you and warmly embrace you. As they do, you feel them, like a body of light, move into you, filling each cell with light, joy, love, health, and energy. Feel the energy as it moves through you—your mind, neck, shoulders, arms, and the palms of your hands—knowing your life *is* in your hands. Down through all organs, tissue, and blood, way down to the bones and down into the mitochondria, the power plants of energy. And way down into your DNA. Ultimate health, energy, and radiant vitality.

Feeling calm yet energized . . . Revitalized and renewed.

Now coming back to room consciousness. Remembering everything you saw and experienced . . . Important remembrances, feelings, and knowings . . . Breathing in a fresh breath of oxygen, vital and energizing . . . Beginning to move your fingers and toes . . . Stretching as you need . . . Feeling light and relaxed in the present . . . your gift of life. Health flowing from the inside out and from the outside in . . . To return to room awareness . . . As you open your eyes, revitalized and radiating life . . .

EMBODY HEALTH, ENERGY, WELLNESS

PURPOSE: *HEALTH, WELLNESS*

SUMMARY: To experience the feelings of health, wellness, energy, and strength.

MY EXPERIENCE: Clients find this imagery inspiring as they experience their future self looking and feeling wonderful. It's a good imagery for those who are feeling stuck in bad habits or an inconsistent health routine.

EXAMPLE: Julie sees her healthy self walking toward her on the beach, looking radiantly healthy. As she gets nearer, she sees that her healthy self is in her best shape ever: strong, vital, eyes shining, with a wide smile. When her healthy self gets close to her, her healthy self says, "Thanks for making me a reality. I feel amazing! Keep it up!" Julie says it reminds her of how incredible she feels when she is actively participating in healthy habits.

ADAPTATION: This imagery can be adapted to strong self, successful self, joyful self, etc. You may add any appropriate wording.

HEALTHY SELF: INSIGHT PAGE QUESTIONS

1. How did you feel meeting your healthy self?
2. Describe the attributes of your healthy self (physical, emotional, mental, spiritual, clothes, overall essence, and attitude).
3. How did you become your healthy self?
4. What else did your healthy self tell you?
5. How did you feel as your healthy self stepped into you and you became your healthy self?
6. How can you use this information in your life to become your ultimate healthy self?

HIGHER POWER / HIGHER SELF

"When you learn to trust in your higher power,
you intuitively understand that you don't have to control everything." ~Anonymous

Getting settled into the surface you're on, closing your eyes. Taking in a long, deep healing breath, inhaling from your stomach up into your chest . . . And releasing it as you let go of all of the day's thoughts and concerns . . . Drifting into a soothing state of serenity . . . Taking in another deep healing breath . . . into the stomach . . . And exhaling anything unlike peace and serenity. Feeling centered, soothed, and content. Breathing in one more deep healing breath . . . into the stomach . . . up into the chest . . . and releasing it . . . as you rest into silent . . . stillness. Your body-mind drifting . . . deep within . . . senses soothed . . .

You sit on a thick, soft blanket on a smooth, flat rock that rests in a pristine meadow in the mountains. The air is so refreshingly clean and you can see for miles below. You feel the gentle warmth of the sun. You hear the soft breeze whispering through the trees and smell the scent of pine. Next to the rock you sit upon is a special tree. You feel a sacred sense of peace within you and all around you, connected with all things.

(Note: Please pause after each question to allow the participant time to visualize and process.)

Slowly, from behind the tree, appears your (Choose Higher Power OR Higher Self).

1. Notice how your Higher Power/Higher Self presents itself to you.
2. How does your Higher Power/Higher Self appear?
3. Feel the qualities of unconditional love and kindness through this being.
4. You are absorbing the feeling of altruistic love from them. You look down and realize that you have a gift for your Higher Power/Higher Self. Give them the gift.
5. How do they respond?
6. Now your Higher Power/Higher Self gives you a gift.
7. What is the gift?
8. And what does it mean to you?
9. Your Higher Power/Higher Self thanks you and gives you important information, direction, or an answer to a question you have at present. Just listen.
10. Thank your Higher Power/Higher Self in any way you choose, knowing that you can always call upon them at any time you need them.

Beginning now to focus your attention on the outside world again, hearing the sounds around you . . . feeling the surface under you . . . Comfortable and content, focused and refreshed. Remembering all you saw and experienced . . . Feeling relaxed, re-centered, and rejuvenated. Beginning to stretch your fingers and toes, counting up one and two, feeling peaceful and content as you return to awareness . . . More aware and alert, three and four . . . beginning to open your eyes, as I say . . . the number five . . . And . . . opening your eyes to the light of the room.

CONNECT WITH HIGHER POWER / HIGHER SELF

PURPOSE: *FAITH, SPIRITUALITY*

SUMMARY: Connect with your Higher Power or Higher Self in a mountain meadow and exchange gifts. *Note: After discussing the meaning of the special tree with participant, you can look it up in the USD for further qualities.*

MY EXPERIENCE: Clients receive inspiration and comfort from this imagery. Clients often visualize spiritual beings from their youth that surprise them. People who say they have no religious or spiritual beliefs connect with their own spirit and with a sense of goodness. People see religious figures, beings of light, goddesses, angels, and shamans that bring insight, or, at the very least, a sense of peace and comfort.

EXAMPLE: Doug sees his Higher Power as Jesus, standing near an olive tree. He feels incredible love and peace standing with Jesus. Jesus gives Doug a cross, and Doug gives Jesus his watch. He says that the cross represents following higher principles, and the watch means that he will give more time to prayer and meditation.

HIGHER POWER/HIGHER SELF: INSIGHT PAGE QUESTIONS

1. How did you feel on the mountaintop?
2. What special tree were you sitting next to?
3. How did your Higher Power/Higher Self appear?
4. How did you feel being in the presence of your Higher Power/Higher Self?
5. What gift did you give to your Higher Power/Higher Self?
6. What gift did your Higher Power/Higher Self give to you?
7. What important information did your Higher Power/Higher Self give you?
8. How can you utilize this to your benefit in your present life?

HORSE

"I call my horses 'divine mirrors'—they reflect back the emotions you put in." ~ Allan Hamilton

Begin to get comfortable as you close your eyes, focus inward, and let go of the day. Take in a deep breath, noticing that any sounds inside or outside simply add to your relaxation. Begin to go to that deep, restful place within yourself: quiet, calm, and centered. Release anything unlike peace as you take in calm with each breath and let go of anything unlike it. Gently, peacefully going to that place within, allowing your entire body-mind to completely relax. Gently moving into the amazing inner landscape of your imagination . . .

You have received a special invitation to a magical horse ranch. You're curious and intrigued after reading their brochure. The brochure explains that the horse ranch is a place where the perfect horse will come to greet you. Even if you have no experience with horses, they have a horse meant just for you and your needs.

When you arrive at the ranch, the sky is wide open and blue. You breathe in the pungent aroma of hay, green grass, and horses. You are told to step out onto a beautiful path that leads you over a small hill to an expansive pasture, where the perfect horse awaits. As you crest the small hill, you see vivid green pastures that expand to the horizon. And there, waiting for you, is the horse . . .

(Note: Please pause after each step to allow the participant time to visualize and process.)

1. Notice the horse's size, color, and any patterns.
2. Observe its face and its eyes.
3. Notice its ears . . . mouth, . . . and mane.
4. What are the horse's qualities?
5. How does the horse respond to you?
6. What would you name this horse?
7. Now have a spontaneous interaction with it.
8. How does it feel interacting with this horse?
9. What do you like about this horse?
10. Is there anything you don't like?
11. Is there anything you would change about it?
12. Is there anything that stands out to you about this horse?
13. Say goodbye to the horse now, knowing you can meet again when you choose.

And now, becoming more aware of the room around you . . . Remembering everything you saw and experienced, coming back as I count up from one to five. Counting up one . . . and two . . . Hearing my voice . . . Hearing sounds in and outside the room . . . Feeling the surface under you . . . Counting up three . . . and four . . . Beginning to stretch your arms and your legs . . . And on the count of five . . . opening your eyes . . . Feeling relaxed, revitalized, and ready for the rest of the day.

TRUST AND OPENNESS

PURPOSE: *RELATIONSHIPS, TRUST*

SUMMARY: Go to a magical horse ranch and meet with a special horse. The interaction between you and the horse can reveal present beliefs relating to trust, love, and relationships and their importance in your life.

MY EXPERIENCE: This imagery can effectively illustrate a client's trust and feelings about intimacy. The distance or closeness between the horse and the person, the horse's actions, and the interaction all give meaningful information on how a person presently relates to love and trust.

EXAMPLE: Teri sees a large, beautiful horse that has the qualities of gentleness and love that make her feel safe. After she pets the horse and enjoys its gentle nature, it rears up and backs away, shaking its head from side to side. She stands still, watching it. The horse gradually comes back to accept and reciprocate her attention. She explains that she recently fell in love, and her partner became frightened and temporarily backed away from their relationship. She said it made her feel unsure and vulnerable, but she learned a lesson by just accepting it and being patient.

HORSE INSIGHT PAGE QUESTIONS

1. Describe the horse's color, size, and patterns.
2. How close did you get to it?
3. What did you see in the horse's eyes?
4. What qualities did the horse possess? What quality stood out to you?
5. How did the horse react to you?
6. What did you name the horse?
7. What did you like about this horse? Was there anything you didn't like?
8. Describe the spontaneous interaction you had with the horse.
9. How did this interaction feel to you?
10. How does this experience relate to your relationships?
11. How can you use this information to improve your relationships?

HOUSE

"Healing means accepting all parts of ourselves, not just the parts we like, but all of us." ~ Louise Hay

Settling into the surface you're on. Closing your eyes as you inhale peace and calm and exhale anything unlike it. And as I count down from five to one, find yourself relaxing more deeply with each word you hear and each sound in or outside. Breathing in, breathing out. Relaxing into peace and calm and the rhythm of the present. Counting down five and four, more and more relaxed, with each beat of your heart and each word you hear me say . . . three and two, deeper into inner contentment. And way down to one, deeply relaxed, journeying inward, into the imagination . . .

And now, you find yourself standing in front of a house.

(Note: Please pause after each question to give the participant time to visualize and process.)

1. Observe the size and architecture of the house. Notice the color, style, and any details.
2. Walk toward the house, open the front door, and step into the living room.
3. Notice the furnishings, colors, and the atmosphere of the room.
4. There is a coffee table with a book on it. Read the title of the book.
5. Continue walking into the dining room. Notice what you see here. Colors, furnishings, and items within.
6. Now enter the kitchen. Look around, observe the style, colors, atmosphere . . . and anything else that catches your attention.
7. Open the refrigerator and look inside. What do you find? Open a cupboard and notice what you see.
8. Now walk into the bedroom. View the furnishings. What are the colors used in the room? What is the atmosphere? How do you feel here?
9. Continue into the bathroom. What colors, items, and details do you notice?
10. Now walk to the stairs and down into the basement. What do you see in the basement? How do you feel in this room?
11. And now you leave the basement and walk to the main floor, then take the stairs up into the attic. What do you see in this attic? What is its condition? How do you feel in this room? Are there any items you notice here?
12. If there is a special item here in the attic, or anywhere else in the house, that seems important to you, you can choose to take it with you.
13. Walk out the back door and take a look at the back of the house. How does it look?
14. Now walk around to the front and look back at the house. If there is anything you'd like to change about it, do that now.

Beginning to return now, remembering everything you saw and experienced . . . As I begin to count up from one to five . . . Counting up one . . . and two . . . Feeling more alert . . . Relaxed and refreshed . . . Breathing in fresh oxygen, feeling more awake and aware . . . stretching your body . . . up three and four . . . Moving your fingers and toes . . . And now, on the count of five . . . opening your eyes . . . refreshed, renewed, and ready for the rest of the day.

EXAMINE ASPECTS OF YOURSELF

PURPOSE: *SELF-DISCOVERY*

SUMMARY: As with all the imageries, do not discuss the meaning of the imagery until after the participant has experienced it. Each room in the house imagery reflects an aspect of the Self. Living room = self; dining room = nurturing others; kitchen = nurturing self; bedroom = rejuvenation, alone time, sexuality; bathroom = release, cleansing; attic = things left behind, superconscious, spirituality; basement = what we suppress or don't want to recognize. *Note: See Dr. Hanscarl Leuner, Chapter 7, (Resources). Find more descriptions regarding the house (colors, etc.) in the USD.*

MY EXPERIENCE: This imagery can elicit great insights. Participant(s) find it valuable to write about the experience for memories sake. For group work, I would use it with no more than four people if you have an hour, due to its length. Most often, clients visualize an imaginary house, and there is an overriding theme. When they imagine a house they have lived in, or are familiar with, they are identifying with the inhabitant(s) of the house or a time in their life that is important. Ask them what is important about this "real" house and what was happening at that time.

EXAMPLE: Ismael sees an open, clean, modern house. The living room (self/present life) is charming. There is a fire burning in the fireplace (warmth). The book on the table is titled Family. The dining room is set for six people with food on the table (nurturing others). Ismael mentions the word *family* often as he describes his imagery. The house is warm and comfortable, until he gets to the basement, where he says, "This room is unfinished." The practitioner asks, "What is unfinished about it?" Ismael responds, "It needs couches, games, and entertainment." He then comments, "I'm planning on getting married soon, and I want a large family, but I'm not ready for the family part yet. I have to get my career on track first."

HOUSE: INSIGHT PAGE QUESTIONS

    1. Describe the house: architecture, color, style, and what you like or don't like about it.

LIVING ROOM

    2. Describe the living room: décor, furniture, colors, the general atmosphere. What sood out?

    3. What was the title of the book you saw? What does it mean to you?

DINING ROOM

    4. Describe the dining room and its contents. How did you feel there?

KITCHEN

    5. Describe the kitchen: atmosphere, colors, appliances, etc. How do you feel in this kitchen?

    6. What was in the refrigerator? And what did you see in the cupboards?

BEDROOM

    7. Describe the bedroom: colors, room, bed, bedding, etc. How do you fell here?

BATHROOM

    8. Describe the bathroom: colors, items, the feel of it . . . What do you like/dislike about this room?

BASEMENT

    9. Describe the basement. What items do you see there? What did you like/dislike?

ATTIC

    10. Describe the attic. How did you feel there? Did you see anything special? If so, what was its meaning to you?

BACK OF HOUSE

    11. Describe the back of the house. How did you feel there? What did you notice?

    12. Did you take an item from the house to keep? If so, what was the importance of this item?

JUDGE

"Self-judgment continues to arise—but the fact that I made a conscious commitment to recognize it has helped me stop feeding the story of being unworthy." ~ Tara Brach

Getting settled into the surface you're on . . . closing your eyes . . . taking in a long, deep healing breath . . . inhaling from your stomach up into your chest . . . and releasing it as you let go of all of the day's thoughts and concerns . . . Just drifting down into a soothing state of serenity . . . Taking in another deep healing breath . . . into the stomach . . . And exhaling anything unlike peace and serenity . . . Feeling centered, soothed, and content . . . Breathing in one more deep healing breath . . . into the stomach . . . up into the chest and releasing it . . . as you rest into the stillness . . . your body and mind drifting deeper into relaxation . . . with all the senses soothed. Drifting deeper, into the imagination, where you find that . . .

You are entering a courtroom to speak on your own behalf. You walk down the center aisle, past the empty gallery toward the judge's bench, and sit in the witness box.

(Note: Please pause after each question to allow the participant time to visualize and process.)

1. As you look at the judge, you see that the judge is another version of you.
2. Look closely at the judge (judgmental you).
3. Does the judge appear to be compassionate and fair?
4. Ask the judge, "What am I accused of?" And listen to the answer.
5. How do you feel about this?
6. Inform the judge that you know you have made mistakes. Many people do.
7. Tell the judge what you have learned.
8. Tell the judge why you deserve the opportunity to change.
9. Tell the judge anything else you feel is important to your future and wellbeing.
10. After hearing what you now know, the judge takes it into account and tells you what should happen next. Listen.
11. What does the judge advise you to do?
12. And how do you feel about that?
13. What will this mean to your future?
14. How will taking this action change your life for the better?

And now, beginning to return . . . Remembering everything you saw and experienced clearly . . . Feeling more alert and focused . . . Beginning to stretch your fingers and toes . . . Feeling balanced and centered . . . Relaxed and refreshed . . . Stretching your body, feeling how the surface under you supports you completely . . . And opening your eyes to the light of the room, renewed and restored . . .

VISUALIZE YOURSELF AS YOUR JUDGE

PURPOSE: *CLARITY, SELF-LOVE*

SUMMARY: Go into a courtroom and see yourself as the judge. Have a dialogue with the judge and speak for yourself, "the accused." Tell the judge what you've learned and how you want to change and improve. The judge gives you direction.

MY EXPERIENCE: Clients can have a hard time with this one! However, it can be very valuable for those who judge themselves harshly. I've had more than one client say, "People say I'm hard on myself, but I never really got it until I saw myself as the judge."

EXAMPLE: James sees himself as a harsh judge. He, as the judge, accuses himself of being selfish and hurting his family. James feels sad and finds it hard to speak for himself. Then James tells the judge that he has come through a lot of pain and learned a lot in the process. He made mistakes, but he has a good heart and loves his family and his life. He needs a chance to show himself and his family who he really is. The judge states that he is willing to give James a chance to prove he can do better, and then he says, "Don't be so stubborn! Listen and learn."

JUDGE: INSIGHT PAGE QUESTIONS

1. Did you feel that the judge would be fair-minded after observing them?
2. What did the judge say you were accused of?
3. How did you feel sitting in the witness stand?
4. What did you tell the judge you had learned?
5. What did you say about deserving a chance?
6. What did the judge tell you was the next step?
7. How will this action change your life for the better?
8. If the judge reminds you of someone in your life who has judged you, who would that be? And are you ready to let their judgments go?
9. What did you learn from this experience?
10. How can you use it for your betterment in the future?

LIBRARY

"I read a book one day and my whole life was changed." ~ Orhan Pamuk

Get into a relaxed position . . . allowing your eyes to close . . . Taking in a deep cleansing breath and releasing it. Allowing yourself to slow down into silence . . . Take in another deep relaxation breath, deep down, into your stomach and up into your chest. Relaxing all muscles from your head, down through your chest, arms, torso, legs, and all the way down into your feet. Filled with soothing serenity . . . so relaxed . . .

And now . . . drifting into the imaginal world where everything is possible. You find yourself at the entrance of a beautiful library. It is warm and inviting and you instinctively know that there are books within this library that will give you greater knowledge and wisdom about yourself.

There are a few people sitting in comfortable chairs near the entrance. You walk toward a ray of light shining down on the aisle straight ahead of you and find that you're in the history section. The light shines down on a book about a time in history that you're very interested in. You see the spine of the book and read the title.

1. What is the title?
2. What about this time in history appeals to you?
3. And how does this relate to your life?

Now you walk over to the biography section.

1. You see a special book that the light shines down on, and you see the name of a person whom you greatly admire on the spine of the book.
2. Who is this person? What qualities or accomplishments do you admire about them?
3. How do those qualities or accomplishments relate to you?

And now you wander down the aisles until you see that you're in the fiction section of the library. You are drawn to a specific genre of fiction.

1. To what section do you go to find this genre?
2. What is it about this type of fiction that interests you?
3. And how does this relate to your life?

Lastly, you head to the self-healing section. There is a book that calls to you, in a bright color.

You step up to the book and take a look at the title on the spine.

1. What is the title of this self-healing book? And how does it relate to you?

And now coming back to room consciousness . . . easily remembering the books . . . on history, fiction, biography, and the self-healing book . . . absorbed and stored . . . Taking in a deep breath, as I count up one and two, informed and educated from within . . . Counting three and four, stretching arms and legs. Stretching fingers and toes. And now, counting up to five, opening your eyes . . . refreshed, renewed, and ready for the rest of the day.

VALUES, GOALS AND INTERESTS

PURPOSE: *SELF-AWARENESS*

SUMMARY: Participant enters a library and chooses books from the history, fiction, biography, and self-healing sections. Describing the importance of these books provides insight into their values and aspirations.

MY EXPERIENCE: This is a good icebreaker imagery with an individual or group to gain knowledge of an individual's interests, goals, and desires. Answering the questions about the books is a reminder and validation for the participant of their own values.

EXAMPLE: Daryl chooses a book from the 1960s about civil rights and says he relates to it because he's interested in improving the world. He chooses a science fiction novel because he's fascinated by futuristic technology. He chooses a biography on Frederick Douglass because of his intelligence and bravery. His self-healing book is titled *You Control Your Life*. He thinks the title is reminding him of his belief that he will achieve his goals.

LIBRARY: INSIGHT PAGE QUESTIONS

1. What book did you choose in the history section? What interests you about this time in history? What do you admire about the people who lived in this time?
2. What book did you choose in the fiction section and why? What is interesting to you about this genre of fiction? What do you find enjoyable about this type of fiction?
3. Whose biography did you choose? What do you admire about this person? What did they accomplish, and what was the theme of their life? How does this relate to you?
4. What was the title of the book you chose in the self-healing section? What does this mean to you? And what actions would you take from it to improve your life?

LIFE'S DREAM INN

"If you can dream it, you can do it." ~ Walt Disney

Getting comfortable now and allowing your eyes to close . . . allowing all your muscles to open and relax . . . letting go, you take in a deep relaxation breath . . . deep down, into your stomach . . . and up into your chest . . . letting that go, along with all the day's thoughts and concerns . . . letting go of anything that isn't right here and right now. Feeling how the surface you're on supports you completely and letting go as you relax into it. All muscles in your body relaxing deeply . . . Hearing the sounds in and outside . . . going within to the imagination, where everything begins and anything is possible . . .

One day as you retrieve your mail from your mailbox, you pull out the most beautiful invitation. It has your name written on it in beautiful writing, and you notice the return address is Life's Dream Inn. When you open the invitation, you find that you've been chosen to visit this magical place. After confirming that this gift is real, the day comes for you to go.

(Note: Please pause after each question to allow the participant to visualize and process.)

You arrive at the Life's Dream Inn. You step out as your luggage is taken and look at the outside. It is as if it was created just for you! Once inside, you look around at the lobby and appreciate the beautiful interior.

1. Notice the colors, decor, the essence.
2. As you begin to check in, the concierge explains that the inn does not use money as currency. You simply offer a gift of value for your life's dream.
3. This gift could be a quality, behavior, belief, or a valued possession that represents your life's dream. You now give your gift to the concierge to enter your life's dream.
4. The concierge thanks you and tells you that there is something important you need for your journey forward. The concierge hands you a gift and might tell you its purpose.
5. Notice what the gift is and what it means to you.
6. Now that you have given and received what you need, the concierge smiles and exclaims, "Welcome to your Life's Dream!" The doors open for you, and you step into your life. How are you using the gift you received from the concierge?
7. And how does the gift you gave support your life's dream?
8. Get a very clear picture of yourself living life fully: healthy, happy, loved, and loving. What do you see yourself doing?
9. How do you feel? What are you doing for work? And leisure?
10. What activities do you do for your health? And how do you look in your dream life?
11. Describe the people around you and their qualities. Imagine that it is the very best it can be with colors very bright and sharp. You feel great joy in your life. What are you giving and what are you receiving?

And now, beginning to return . . . Remembering everything you saw and experienced clearly . . . As I begin to count up from one to five . . . Counting up one . . . and two . . . Feeling more alert . . . Relaxed and refreshed from this journey within . . . Up three and four . . . Beginning to stretch your fingers and toes . . . Feeling great . . . And opening your eyes on the count of five.

LIVE YOUR LIFE'S DREAM

PURPOSE: *INSPIRATION*

SUMMARY: Give and receive what you need for your life's dream. Experience yourself living your life's dream.

MY EXPERIENCE: Participants enjoy being whisked off to a beautiful inn created to their liking. They are reminded of what is truly important to them and which people and activities add to their most fulfilling life.

EXAMPLE: Darnella arrives at the Life's Dream Inn, which is a large rustic hotel up in the mountains. She gives the concierge a red glass heart, which represents her love for life, and the concierge gives her a compass, which she says represents direction. Darnella sees herself meditating and working out for her health and spending time with good friends and family. She visualizes finishing her degree, teaching, traveling, and meeting new and interesting people for fun and relaxation.

ADAPTATIONS: This imagery can be adapted to sobriety (what you give and receive for it), or any other conditions such as health, happiness, peace, joy, success, etc.

LIFE'S DREAM INN: INSIGHT PAGE QUESTIONS

1. Describe the Life's Dream Inn.
2. Was there anything this place reminded you of?
3. What gift did you give the concierge for your life's dream?
4. What did the concierge give you? What meaning do these gifts have?
5. When you walked out into your life's dream, what did you experience?
6. Were there other people there? If so, who were they and what do they mean to you?
7. What activities did you see yourself doing for your health?
8. What work were you doing? What for fun and leisure?
9. How were you using the gift that the concierge gave you for your journey?
10. How did living your best life feel?
11. How can you best use this information to create your life's dream?

MASQUERADE

"Love has a powerful way of removing the mask we all insist on wearing." ~ Jessy

Begin to get comfortable as you close your eyes, focus inward, and let go of the day. Take in a deep breath, noticing that any sounds in or outside simply add to your relaxation. Begin to go to that deep, restful place within you: quiet, calm, and centered. Take in peace and calm with each breath and release anything unlike it as you exhale. Gently, peacefully going to that place within, allowing your entire body-mind to completely relax. Relax, as you move into that magical inner landscape of your imagination . . .

It is a cool, starry night. You have been invited to a masquerade ball. You are dressed and ready to go. Before you walk out of the door to leave, you pick your mask up off the table and take a moment to examine it.

(Note: Please pause after each question to allow the participant time to visualize and process.)

1. What does the mask look like?
2. What color or colors is the mask?
3. What is it made of? What is its texture?
4. Notice small details . . . What do you like about it? . . . Is there anything you don't like?
5. You are now transported to the masquerade. You walk into the room with your mask on.
6. Notice what you're wearing and how you feel as you enter the masquerade.
7. How do people respond to you?
8. What does your mask hide? And what does it project? What would you name your mask?
9. Halfway through the masquerade, the host announces that you can choose to turn your mask inside out. You take your mask off and turn it inside out.
10. What does the inside of the mask look like? Notice the details. Do you like the inside?
11. Is there anything you don't like about it? What would you name the inside of the mask?
12. You choose either to wear the mask inside out or as it was before. If you chose to change it, how did you feel wearing it inside out?
13. And how is this different from before?
14. Now the host announces that you may take off your mask if you choose. If you choose to continue the masquerade without your mask, how do you feel without it?
15. As the night goes on and the masquerade comes to an end, what would you like to do with the mask?

And now, beginning to return . . . Clearly remembering everything you saw and experienced. Feeling more alert . . . Relaxed and refreshed. Hearing the sound of my voice, becoming more aware of the surface under you, beginning to stretch your fingers and toes . . . Returning to awareness . . . And now opening your eyes to the light of the room, renewed and ready for the rest of the day.

THE MASK YOU WEAR

PURPOSE: *SELF-AWARENESS*

SUMMARY: Go to a masquerade ball. Inspect your mask inside and out. Understand what you might cover up or what you wish to project and what your inner mask represents. ***Note:*** *After receiving information from the participant on the meaning of their mask, you can gain further information about color, texture, etc. from the Universal Symbol Dictionary.*

MY EXPERIENCE: Clients enjoy this imagery and receive insight about showing their authenticity or projecting another image. Many participants find that the mask is hiding their vulnerabilities or projecting a quality they feel they lack. There is insight gained from how they feel about the inside of their mask and whether they choose to take the mask off or keep it on.

EXAMPLE: Pam sees herself wearing a black and green mask with translucent sequins on it. She is wearing a flowy black dress with high-heeled boots to the masquerade. She feels mysterious and flirtatious as she walks into the crowd. Halfway through the masquerade, she chooses to turn her mask inside out. On the inside, she sees soft sage green material, which represents her soft natural side and love of the earth. She feels this is her authentic self, yet she feels her mask isn't hiding anything. She realizes that she's more confident than she sometimes acknowledges. She feels the name of the mask she uses in the world would be *Serene*. Pam says she presents herself as calm, and people say she is "chill" even when she's feeling anxious on the inside. She would name her inner mask *Earthy*.

MASQUERADE: INSIGHT PAGE QUESTIONS

1. Describe your mask. What was it made of? Its texture? Color? Any other distinctions?
2. What did you like about the mask? Was there anything you didn't like?
3. How did you feel as you walked into the masquerade with your clothing and mask? What did you notice about the other masqueraders? How did they react (if they did) to you?
4. What did the mask hide? What did it project? What did you name the mask?
5. Describe the inside of the mask. Did you like it? Was there anything you disliked about it? If you chose to wear it inside out, how did this change how you felt about yourself and your interaction with others?
6. What would you name the *inside* of the mask?
7. When given the opportunity to take the mask off completely, what did you do?
8. How did you feel if you chose to go without the mask? How was this different than wearing it?
9. What did the mask give to you? What did the mask hide?
10. How did the mask limit you, if it did?
11. If you had a name for the mask you wear out in the world, what would you call it?

MOUNTAIN

"You keep putting one foot in front of the other,
and then one day you look back and you've climbed a mountain." ~ Tom Hiddleston

Get settled into the surface you're on, close your eyes, and take in a long, deep healing breath. Inhale from your stomach up into your chest, and release it as you let go of all of the day's thoughts and concerns . . . Drift down into a soothing state of serenity . . . Take in another deep healing breath . . . into the stomach . . . and exhale anything unlike peace and calm. Feel centered, soothed, and content . . . breathe in one more deep healing breath . . . into the stomach . . . up into the chest, and release it . . . as you rest into the stillness . . . your body and mind drift deeper . . . within . . . into relaxation . . . with all the senses soothed . . . drift deeper . . . into the imagination, to find that . . .

You are driving toward a mountain that you plan to climb. You stop the car, get out, and take a picture of the mountain from a distance.

1. Describe the mountain.
2. Now you arrive and stand at the base of the mountain. How do you feel about your upcoming ascent?
3. How does the path look as you begin walking upward?
4. How steep is the path, and how do feel on it?
5. You continue your ascent. What terrain do you encounter?
6. Notice your energy level.
7. Now you come upon a challenge. What is the challenge you face?
8. How do you work through it, and how difficult was it?
9. What do you notice around you as you continue to walk upward?
10. Now you arrive at the summit of the mountain. How does it feel at the top? And what do you see in the distance?
11. You enjoy the vista for a time, and then you hear a voice, saying your name.
12. You turn to see a Wise One, with eyes twinkling with love, intelligence, and warmth. You feel an aura of kind wisdom emanating from them.
13. Ask the Wise One their name and greet them in whatever way you feel is appropriate.
14. The Wise One tells you that they are aware of your recent progress, and have a gift for you for your continued journey. What is the gift? And how can you use this in the future?
15. Now the Wise One gives you a message to ponder. The Wise One asks you "What can you do to create more joy and fulfillment through your continued goals?"

Now thank the Wise One in whatever way you choose and say goodbye for now, knowing you can always speak to them again as you need.

And now, beginning to return to room consciousness . . . Beginning to become more aware as you pay attention to your breath . . . Hearing my words and the sounds in and outside . . . With each word I say . . . and each breath you take in . . . And release . . . becoming more aware of the outer world. Beginning to stretch your arms and legs and take in a refreshing breath, feeling more alert . . . Hearing the sound of my voice . . . Remembering everything you saw and experienced clearly. Wiggling your fingers and toes . . . And now, gently, opening your eyes, rejuvenated and revitalized . . . and ready for the rest of the day.

HOW YOU RISE ABOVE CHALLENGES

PURPOSE: *SELF-AWARENESS, MOTIVATION*

SUMMARY: Connect with a Wise One at the summit of the mountain path. Receive information and a gift for your present life journey. Have a spontaneous vision regarding this issue.

MY EXPERIENCE: Clients usually find this imagery comforting as well as inspiring. They sometimes see relatives (grandparents, aunts, or uncles) as the Wise One.

EXAMPLE: Jeff sees a wise old man with gray hair and twinkling brown eyes, who feels kind, wise, and loving. The old man says his name is Walter and grins. Jeff notices a gentle humor that he appreciates in Walter. Walter tells Jeff he needs to "Take care of business." Walter then winks and says, "You know what to do—just get into action." He shows him a vision in which Jeff is happy and at peace after taking care of some business he's been putting off. Jeff takes the suggestion well since it is not demanding but suggestive and intuitive.

MOUNTAIN: INSIGHT PAGE QUESTIONS

1. Describe the mountain.
2. How did you feel about the climb up as you stood at the base of the mountain?
3. Describe the path. What terrain did you encounter?
4. How was the ascent and your energy level?
5. What challenge did you come upon?
6. How did you transcend the challenge?
7. Did the journey become easier or more difficult as you climbed?
8. What did you see in the distance?
9. Describe the Wise One you met at the top. What was their name?
10. What gift did they gave you for your future journeys?
11. What does it mean to you? And how can you use it in the future?
12. What can you do in the future to bring more joy and fulfillment?

POWER SOURCE

"Our authentic power is found in our truth. This is the place that shows us how to give what is so very good about ourselves." ~ Jeanne McElvaney

Getting settled into the surface you're on, closing your eyes . . . Taking in a long, deep healing breath, inhaling from your stomach up into your chest, and releasing it as you let go of all of the day's thoughts and concerns . . . Drifting down into a soothing state of serenity . . . Taking in another healing breath . . . into the stomach . . . Exhaling anything unlike peace and serenity. Resting into the stillness . . . Your body and mind drifting deeper . . . into relaxation . . . with all the senses soothed . . . Drifting deep . . . into the imagination . . . into an open field with a blue sky above you. Knowing that in the imagination, we can do anything . . .

(Note: Please pause after each step to allow the participant time to visualize and process.)

You see your mother standing in front of you. She has an electric outlet in her stomach, and you notice that you have an electrical cord with a plug on it coming from your stomach.

1. You connect the cord into your mother's / father's stomach and feel their energy flowing into your body.
2. What kind of energy do you receive from them?
3. How does it feel? And what is happening in your body?
4. Is there a place in your body you feel it more than others?
5. Now unplug from their energy and tell them about the energy you received from them.
6. How do you use this energy to benefit you (and possibly others) in your present life?
7. Tell them about the supportive energy you received.
8. And what about any other type of energy you received? How does that feel in your body?
9. How do you use this energy in your present life?
10. Now thank them for what this has taught you.
11. And allow the image of your mother / father to fade away.

Now you see your father standing in front of you. (Repeat above with father.)

And now, you notice that standing in front of you is your own body of light, your own unlimited energy source. The gift *to* and *of* you. See it glowing with energy. It is *beautiful*. You stand up and step into it.

1. What is happening in your body?
2. Let your own energy flow through you and embody it. Feel it all the way down to your bones, deep into the DNA of you. Feel the vibration of your own life, of your own power.
3. Thank your unlimited power source, feel its energy, and feel it within you as you return. Know that in reality, it is the essence of you, and you can acknowledge it, be aware of it, and use it any time you choose.

Now coming back to room consciousness, feeling relaxed and renewed, counting up one and two, feeling more aware . . . Refreshed and refocused. Feeling the surface under you, any sounds around you. Three. Feeling at peace, in harmony, at one. Four and up to five . . . And opening your eyes . . . revitalized. Feeling grounded, empowered, and ready for the rest of the day!

EMBODY YOUR OWN POWER

PURPOSE: *CONFIDENCE*

SUMMARY: Experience the energy you received from your mother and father. Feel what was supportive or challenging about their energy and what you learned from it. Then experience your own power/energy source.

MY EXPERIENCE: This can be an insightful imagery regarding parental influence and one's personal independence. It can bring tears of joy or sorrow. It connects clients to their somatic reactions to parents and to more awareness on how it can limit or improve their lives.

EXAMPLE: Mitch felt love and understanding from his mother, as well as anxiety. He felt ambition and drive from his father, along with judgment. He learned from his mother that you can't let worry hold you back. Through his father's judgment, he learned to be less judgmental. When he felt his own energy, he was surprised at how freeing it felt and realized that he is feeling more independent and more "himself" at present.

POWER SOURCE: INSIGHT PAGE QUESTIONS

MOTHER

1. Describe the power you received from your mother.
2. How did it feel in your body?
3. Was there a place in your body that felt more energy than others? If so, where?
4. Describe what felt unsupportive about this energy.
5. Describe what felt supportive about the energy.
6. What have you learned from this energy, and how can you use this to benefit your present life?

FATHER:

1. Describe the power you received from your father.
2. How did it feel in your body?
3. Was there a place in your body that felt more energy than others? If so, where?
4. Describe what felt unsupportive about this energy.
5. And what felt supportive about this energy?
6. What have you learned from this energy, and how can you use this to benefit your present life?

SELF:

1. How did your own unlimited power source feel in your body?
2. Was there a place in your body you felt it more than others? If so, where?
3. Describe what was positive about this energy. Any negative energy?
4. What have you learned from this energy, and how can you use this energy to benefit your present life?

PURPOSE

"There is no greater gift you can give or receive than to honor your calling. It's why you were born. And how you become the most truly alive." ~ Oprah Winfrey

Rest into the surface you're on . . . Letting go of anything from the day. Closing your eyes as you take in a deep healing breath . . . Relaxing into the present . . . Slowing down, taking another healing breath and releasing it. Gently breathing into your stomach and up into your chest and exhaling. Giving yourself complete permission to relax and rest into the stillness of the moment . . . Into your center, in the here and now. Gently breathe in and out . . . as your breathing slows down. Drifting down to observe and absorb the quiet . . . in the center . . . of the soothing . . . silence . . . within . . . Moving into the imagination . . .

You are in the middle of the most beautiful meadow. It's vibrantly green and full of life. You smell the fresh, pungent scent of the earth and see and hear the grass swaying around you. Flowers of vivid colors blow gently in the breeze. The air moves softly over your skin. Everything is flourishing. You feel alive, open, and full of possibilities. Up above, white clouds move so slowly through the bluest sky you've ever seen . . . so beautiful . . . peaceful . . . and serene.

You're walking on a path through the middle of this meadow. The path begins to curve to the right. You follow it until ahead you see a small hill and see that the path you're on goes straight up to the top. As you reach the base of the hill, you look up to see an image at the top of the hill that represents your purpose.

(Note: Please pause after each step to allow the participant time to visualize and process.)

1. What is the image?
2. And now, you begin walking up the hill to your purpose.
3. On both sides of the path, you feel the presence of things that might try to divert you from reaching the top . . . but they cannot. There is something that keeps them from distracting you. As you pass these distractions, notice what they are and what keeps the distractions at bay.
4. What is it that the distractions keep you from doing?
5. Experience your clear intention as you proceed up the path. Feel the strength of your intention, aware of the power in your body and legs as you place one foot in front of the other, stepping up, moving upward, one step at a time.
6. And now, you reach the top. Notice the image that represents your purpose.
7. Observe it closely. Notice the clarity, details, and colors.
8. You can walk around it to see it very clearly, and you can even look down on it from above.
9. And now . . . step into the image and become it.
10. How does it feel to experience your purpose? (ample pause)

Enjoy it now, knowing that you embody your purpose each day as it manifests through your intentions, actions, and behavior.

And now, beginning to return . . . Remembering everything you saw and experienced clearly . . . As I begin to count up from one to five . . . Counting up one . . . and two . . . Feeling more alert . . . relaxed and refreshed . . . Up three, positive with possibilities . . . And four . . . beginning to stretch your fingers and toes . . . feeling inspired . . . And opening your eyes on the count of five. Revitalized and ready for the rest of the day!

EMBODY YOUR PURPOSE

PURPOSE: *INSPIRATION, MOTIVATION*

SUMMARY: See a symbol that represents your purpose at the top of a small hill. Walk up the hill toward your purpose and notice the distractions on each side of you while not allowing them to keep you from progressing. Feel your power and intention that take you to the top. Reach your purpose, step into it, and embody it. *Note: As with other imageries, after fully discussing the participant's interpretation of imagery, you can look up a symbol's meaning, color, etc. in the Universal Symbol Dictionary.*

MY EXPERIENCE: My clients and students gain a lot from this imagery. It clarifies their distractions and fears, they enjoy experiencing the attainment of their purpose and it inspires motivation.

EXAMPLE: Rozanne sees herself at the top of the hill working in a new career. As she walks upward, she hears people's criticism, which gets her attention. She also feels her strong intention, and she arrives at the top of the hill. She joins the vision of herself working with another person one-on-one. She feels satisfied, gratified, and joyful in her purpose. She says it reminds her once more to "Keep doing the work; and let go and let God."

ADAPTATION: You can adapt this imagery to anything goal-oriented such as ultimate health, love, joy, peace, balance, success in career, relationships, financial abundance, etc.

PURPOSE: INSIGHT PAGE QUESTIONS

1. What image at the top of the hill represented your purpose?
2. What were the distractions on each side of the path going up the hill?
3. And what was it that it, or they, could limit you from doing?
4. How did you feel about the distractions?
5. What was it that kept the distractions from influencing your upward climb?
6. How did it feel walking up the hill, experiencing yourself as clear purpose?
7. When you reached the top, how did the image of your purpose look?
8. How did it feel to be close to your purpose?
9. How did it feel when you became it?
10. How can you utilize this experience to assist you in attaining or maintaining your purpose?

RAIN

"Life is like a rainbow; you need both the sun and rain to make its colors appear." ~ Anonymous

Relaxing now, taking in a deep breath . . . inhaling into your stomach . . . and up into your chest . . . And letting that go, along with all the day's thoughts and concerns . . . letting go of anything that isn't right here and right now. Noticing how the surface you're on supports you completely . . . letting all the muscles in your body relax into gravity. Hearing the sounds in and outside . . . enjoying this moment of complete quiet, feeling at peace, listening to the stillness . . . in the center of the silence. And now going within and imagining that . . .

You sit comfortably under a covered porch at a cabin in the woods. As you look out at the forest opening, you see raindrops beginning to fall slowly in syncopated rhythm. You inhale the moist air, heavy with the cleansing scents of earth and rain. The low dark clouds move slowly over the forest as the rain begins to fall in a steady shower. As you lie back in your comfortable chair on the covered porch, you close your eyes and listen to the patter on the roof as it lulls you into a lovely relaxation on this lazy, languorous day . . . Relaxing so deeply . . .

And as you rest, a symbol appears that represents cleansing and renewal.

(Note: Please pause after each step to allow the participant time to visualize and process.)

1. Just allow the symbol to appear in front of you, letting it be what it is.
2. What *is* the symbol?
3. Notice its size . . . and its shape. What color is the symbol?
4. The symbol has a message for you about cleansing and renewal. Just listen . . . you might hear it, or just intuitively know it.
5. Thank the symbol for its message, and take it within you to just the right place, where it reminds and refreshes you whenever needed.

Feeling safe and centered in the forest, hearing the soothing sound of the steady rain, you breathe in the cleansing fragrance of pine and know that you're safe and sound.

The drizzle slows, the earth cleansed and steeped in nourishment. You smell the fresh scent of rain mixed with earth. Rays of sunlight shine down through dispersing clouds, shedding light upon the forest. The rain droplets, heavy on the leaves of trees, shine under the sunlight. Like the trees, you've grown stronger through storms, able to nourish yourself and others. Bathed in the warmth of the sun, renewed and refreshed, feeling cleansed and new.

Now, returning to the gift of the present. Remembering what you saw and experienced . . . Breathing in freshness . . . Beginning to move your fingers and toes . . . Stretching as you need . . . Feeling light and relaxed in the here and now . . . Returning to room awareness . . . Lighter and brighter . . . Stretching your arms and legs . . . and opening your eyes . . . to the light of the room . . . refreshed and renewed.

CLEANSING AND RENEWAL

PURPOSE: *BEING PRESENT*

SUMMARY: Watch the rain as you rest on a cabin porch in the forest. Visualize a symbol that represents cleansing and renewal. Take the symbol within to embody it.

MY EXPERIENCE: This is a calming, relaxing, and reassuring imagery. A good one for anxious participants needing physical and emotional relaxation.

EXAMPLE: Ryan enjoys watching the rain and is grateful that he's able to relax in this beautiful place. He sees a fish that represents cleansing and renewal. He knows that it was fishing and the quiet of nature that helped cleanse and renew him. He feels proud of himself and the life he's created, and he knows he can let go of the past to enjoy the present.

RAIN: INSIGHT PAGE QUESTIONS

1. How did it feel watching the rain as you rested on the porch?
2. Describe the symbol that represented cleansing and renewal.
3. What message did the symbol give you?
4. What does it mean to you?
5. Where did you place it in your body?
6. And what made you decide to place it there?
7. How did you feel embodying the symbol of cleansing and renewal?
8. How can you use this in the future to refresh and renew your energy?

RETURN TO THE FUTURE

"Caring for your inner child has a powerful and surprisingly quick result.
Do it, and the child heals." ~ Martha Beck

Getting comfortable now, closing your eyes . . . Taking in a deep healing breath, inhaling from your stomach up into your chest, and releasing it as you let go of all of the day's thoughts and concerns . . . Drifting down into a soothing state of serenity . . . Taking in another deep healing breath . . . And exhaling anything unlike peace and serenity . . . Feeling centered, soothed, and serene . . . Breathing in one more deep healing breath . . . Up into the chest . . . releasing it . . . resting into the stillness . . . Body and mind drifting deeper . . . into relaxation . . . All senses soothed . . . Drifting deeper . . . into the imagination . . .

(Note: Please pause after each question to allow participant to visualize and process.)

And now, softly, safely, gently going back in time . . . You find that you are with your ten-year-old self.

1. What do they look like? What are they wearing?
2. How does your ten-year-old self respond to you?
3. Greet them in whatever way you choose. If they don't know who you are, let them know.
4. What do you feel for this child? Send them all your love and comfort them if you feel they need it.
5. How do they respond? . . . Ask the child what they need.
6. Are you able to give them this? Now tell them all the good qualities they possess.
7. And tell the child anything else you would like to say.

Now invite them to come with you to visit their future. Take their hand and walk them into your present home. Let them explore. How do they respond to your home? How is this home different from their home at ten years old? If you choose, introduce them to your loved ones. *(Allow an ample pause.)*

How do they feel about these people?

Now, if you choose, take your ten-year-old self to watch you as you do your present work.

8. What do they think about this work you do? Allow them to do whatever they choose now.
9. After they have enjoyed that, embrace them again, feeling their essence. What do they understand now that they didn't understand before?
10. And how can you use this in your present life?

And now as you hold them, allow them to integrate into you, like a body of light, that now has new knowledge and wisdom. The essence of this new ten-year-old melds into you, brightening your mind, behind your eyes and down through your body: your heart, lungs, stomach, and abdomen. Down through your legs, moving you forward with new understanding, purpose, and energy.

And now, returning to room consciousness . . . Hearing my words, the sounds in and outside . . . With each word I say . . . and each breath you take in and release . . . more aware of the outer world. Beginning to stretch your arms and legs. Taking in a deeper breath, feeling more alert . . . Hearing the sound of my voice, remembering everything you saw and experienced clearly . . . And now . . . gently . . . opening your eyes . . . refreshed and revitalized . . . and ready for the rest of the day.

HEALING INNER CHILD

PURPOSE: *INNER CHILD*

CAVEAT: If the participant's present life is traumatic, skip this imagery. If their life is not optimal, the child will sometimes give the participant important information on what changes are needed.

SUMMARY: Revisit one's ten-year-old self. Dialogue with the child, asking their needs and giving them support. Bring the child to one's present home to meet family/loved ones and/or to your workplace (if working outside the home). Child experiences the participant's present life and receives a new perspective.

MY EXPERIENCE: This imagery is powerful to reframe and re-inform one's inner child of what has changed. Often, the adult has information to help the child understand and heal. However, as in the caveat above, sometimes the child has information for the adult. In either case, this can be an enlightening imagery.

EXAMPLE: Juan is financially successful, in his fifties, and suffering from executive burnout. He visits his ten-year-old self and softly cries as he sees the ten-year-old fishing in a beautiful stream, relaxed and content. He takes his ten-year-old self to his luxurious home. His ten-year-old self is amazed and impressed. He takes his ten-year-old self to work. The child is shocked at the responsibility his adult self has. Juan, crying, feels the loss of time, innocence, and simplicity in his life. His ten-year-old self tells him that he just wants to fish. After the imagery, Juan says that he knows he desperately needs greater peace and intends to create more leisure for himself in the future, whatever it takes.

RETURN TO THE FUTURE: INSIGHT PAGE QUESTIONS

1. Describe your ten-year-old self and their emotional state. What did they wear?
2. How did you feel about this child?
3. What did the child tell you they needed? Can you give them this?
4. What did you tell the child? What good qualities did you tell them they possessed?
5. How did they respond to your present home?
6. If you introduced them to loved ones, how did they respond?
7. How did they respond to watching you work?
8. What do they now understand better than they did then?
9. What was the result of the ten-year-old seeing their future?
10. What has changed in the years since childhood?
11. How have your values changed?
12. How can you use this to help you in the present?

RIVER

"Go with the flow. Take the path of no resistance.
Be like the river, live your life in the flow." ~Anonymous

You're in a small, comfortable boat, resting back into a comfy seat . . . floating down a slow-moving river . . . at just the perfect pace for you. Leisurely drifting under canopied trees, translucent green, under the sun. Rays of light stream down through the trees . . . and the sunlight dapples on the water, as you slowly flow with the river . . . You hear the lapping of the water against the riverbanks as you float so smoothly with the river. Smell the cleansing scent of water . . . and the musky fragrance of earth. Feel the cooling sensation of the water flowing under you . . . as you float gently past trees and green landscapes on this lazy day. Water, flowing, just like the life that flows through you . . . Wide open and peaceful. Flowing with ease. Slow . . . smooth and comfortable. Floating . . . as the sunlight glints and sparkles on the flowing water.

Letting go . . . letting your mind drift. Letting the world take care of itself. Breathing in the fresh coolness of water, the earthy fragrance of tree bark, and the clean scent of plants and trees surrounding you. And as you float in your mind and body, and relax even deeper . . . the river widens, slows, and opens up into the most exquisitely peaceful lake, where you can just *relax* on still water, listening to the sounds of the trees rustling in the softest breeze. A calm slowing down . . . as relaxation continues, deepens, and becomes part of you . . .

1. The trees above whisper a word or phrase to you . . . to remember and remind you . . . of this deep relaxation . . .
2. That you can remember any time . . . anywhere . . .
3. A word or phrase . . . to repeat in your mind . . . as you breathe in the air . . . Anytime . . . anywhere . . .
4. Breathe in the air, anytime, anywhere . . . say the word . . . and . . . *Ree-lax* . . .

As you say your word or phrase to yourself and anchor in this beautiful place of freedom . . . Feeling the gentle rocking of the boat on the water . . . and the lapping of the water against the boat . . . lulling you into deeper relaxation. The sun warms your body as the lake gently laps against the shore . . . in that timeless way . . . that just goes on . . . and on . . . forever . . . and ever. Leaving everything behind . . . feeling loose and relaxed . . . safe and comfortable. With the calm, quiet water surrounding you . . . letting go . . . into contentment . . . into the soothing stillness within . . . So relaxed . . . with blues and greens . . . scents and scenes . . . that lull you . . . gently . . . floating in freedom. Refreshed and so relaxed.

Now beginning to return to room consciousness, feeling more aware and relaxed. Trusting that remembrances of now remain . . . Remembering to forget or forgetting to remember what is past . . . To remain . . . in the now . . . right now . . . relaxed . . . To receive the gift of life. Counting up one and two . . . More aware of the surface under you . . . supporting you completely . . . Counting three and four . . . Moving fingers and toes . . . Beginning to stretch your body . . . And upon the count of five, returning . . . relaxed and rejuvenated . . . Aware and alert . . . Opening your eyes into the here . . . and the now.

ANCHOR IN RELAXATION RESPONSE

PURPOSE: *BEING PRESENT*

SUMMARY: Relax as you float down a slow-moving river that flows into a lake. Relax into present time and receive a word or phrase to use to relax whenever needed.

MY EXPERIENCE: This imagery offers the participant the self-soothing tool of an *anchor* to the feeling-state of relaxation, which they can use outside the imagery experience. Good when an individual client or group has had a busy day and simply needs to relax.

EXAMPLE: Within the imagery, Jerry sees himself floating down the river, but he has thoughts from the day that interrupt his relaxation. He notices his shoulders are tight. As he continues to allow himself to relax into his imagination and engage his senses, he begins to enjoy the experience. He hears the words "slow down" to remember the deep relaxation he is feeling and to trust that he can intentionally relax naturally by using this phrase with his breath when he chooses.

RIVER INSIGHT PAGE QUESTIONS

1. What did you notice as you began floating down the river?
2. What changed as you continued to let go and flow with the river?
3. At what point did you forget about the outside world and relax into your imagination?
4. How did it feel floating on the still water in the lake?
5. What word or phrase came to you to use with your breath to remember to embody this relaxation?
6. Where and when can you use this to help yourself relax?

ROOM REPRESENTING

"The world as we have created it is a process of our thinking.
It cannot be changed without changing our thinking." ~ Albert Einstein

Note: Room Representing can represent emotions or challenges such as anxiety, fear, guilt, shame, addiction, codependency, confusion, etc.

Settling into the surface you're on . . . Letting your body completely relax into gravity. Closing your eyes as you take in a deep, healing breath . . . Allowing all of your muscles to expand and let go . . . Slowing down . . . Taking another healing breath in and releasing it . . . Gently breathing into your stomach and up into your chest, and exhaling. Giving yourself permission to completely relax and rest in the stillness of the moment . . . into your center, in the here and now. Gently breathing in and out, out and in, as your breathing becomes slower . . . Shifting your attention inward, into the center of calm and contentment. Your mind and body at peace, as you move deeper into that center to allow yourself to wonder and wander . . . Drifting down to observe and absorb the quiet . . . in the center . . . of the soothing . . . silence . . . within . . . and now, going into the imagination.

You are opening the door to a room. This room is called the Room of (insert emotion, challenge, or situation here). You are safe to enter the room, as you have all the power, in your imagination.

(Note: Please pause after each step to allow the participant time to visualize and process.)

1. Notice how the room looks.
2. Look around; observe the contents and the energy of the room.
3. What do you like in this room?
4. And what items or aspects don't you like?
5. How do you feel being in this room?
6. You are now free to change the room in whatever way you choose.
7. Remove whatever creates the (*emotion, challenge, or situation*).
8. You can change anything you want about this room; the walls, windows, furnishings, floor, anything at all; whatever brings greater peace to you. (*Give ample pause.*)
9. How does the room look now?
10. And what would be a more appropriate name for this redesigned room?

And now, begin to focus your attention on the outside world again, as you hear the sounds around you . . . Feeling the surface under you . . . Feeling comfortable and content, focused, and refreshed. Remembering everything you saw and experienced . . . Beginning to stretch your fingers and toes, counting up one and two, feeling at peace as you return to awareness . . . More aware and alert, three and four . . . And on the count of five, opening your eyes, as I say . . . the number . . . five. Feeling relaxed, recentered and rejuvenated.

REARRANGE A ROOM REPRESENTING CHALLENGE

PURPOSE: *SELF-DISCOVERY*

SUMMARY: Walk into a room that represents an emotion or challenge. Experience the feelings in the room; notice its contents and what creates and amplifies the emotion or challenge. Redesign the room. Remove what you choose and add what creates greater peace or balance. *Note: After discussing what the participant's meanings of the room are, you can check in the Universal Symbol Dictionary for further information on any details in the room.*

MY EXPERIENCE: This is a great imagery to help clients clarify what contributes to their emotions or challenge and what to release. It can also inspire and empower them to move toward needed change.

EXAMPLE: Rita walks into a room representing anxiety. The room is noisy, with bright lights and too many people. She says it reminds her of a very busy restaurant. Rita says she feels trapped and anxious. When she redesigned the room, she took all but one person out and added furniture so it looked like a comfortable living room. She explained that her job forces her to travel often and socialize with strangers, and her job is making her anxiety worse. She has been considering changing her career to something less stressful and more meaningful, and the imagery reinforced this idea.

ROOM REPRESENTING: INSIGHT PAGE QUESTIONS

1. How did you feel walking into the room called (whatever their challenge was)?
2. Describe the room. What size was it? What color? Were there windows, pictures, furniture? Any other items?
3. What did you notice in the room that added to the feeling of (the challenge)?
4. What did you choose to remove from the room?
5. How did you change it/redesign it?
6. And how did it look and feel when it was changed?
7. How do these changes relate to your present life?
8. What more appropriate name did you give the room?
9. How can you utilize this information to help you?

STARS

"The total number of stars in the universe is larger than all the grains of sand
on all the beaches of the planet Earth." ~ Carl Sagan

You're sitting on the most beautiful beach just after sunset . . . Your feet are relaxed in the warm, white sand . . . You take in a breath of the fresh scent of the sea . . . The sun sparkles off the water like diamonds . . . You hear the sound of the surf . . . that quiet roar . . . that disappears into silence. The palm trees rustle in the breeze . . . so relaxed . . . so at peace. Allowing the misty scent of salt in the air and the soothing sounds to lull you deeper into a wonderful relaxation . . . and into the imagination, where everything is possible . . .

You take a handful of soft, silky sand and let it sift through your fingers. You watch the tiny grains fall back onto the shore you rest upon. Limitless sand, like stars in the sky. You look at the horizon; at that imaginary line between the sea and sky that really isn't there. Knowing it's all relative, just perspective. Rising above it, expanding your view, the line becomes a curve, and the curve becomes a circle. The circle of the earth, the sun and moon, and out into the galaxy: one hundred billion stars, ten trillion galaxies . . . ever creating . . . and expanding.

And the sky begins to darken. Starlight from millions of years past begins to gift you with its gentle glow. And you wonder at the wonder of this ever-changing, evolving universe that you're a part of. From the smallest to the largest, all here for you . . . the shore supporting your body, the air you inhale and exhale, all connected to the universe around you, a part of you.

The sky begins to turn velvety black. The stars brighten and twinkle. You connect with one star that begins to enlarge, close enough to touch. You reach up and take it in your hands and feel it, alive with cosmic energy. Every cell of your body, made up of the same stuff as the stars. All the creative energy within you, body, mind, and soul.

(Note: Please pause after each step to allow the participant time to visualize and process.)

See the bright glow shimmering and shining within you . . . Knowing all things are illuminated, becoming, you see a symbol form within this light. This symbol represents abundance, creation, expansion.

1. What is the symbol?
2. Begin to walk around it. Look at it from all sides. Now, join with it to feel its energy.
3. How does it feel to be expansive, dynamic, bursting with creative promise and growth?
4. Everything is a possibility . . . Endless like this universe, always giving of itself. Creation flowing through and from it. You . . . creation . . . creating. Ask the symbol . . .
5. What is the most important thing I am to create?
6. Get a picture of your creation and hold it in your mind. A clear, vivid, colorful picture in your mind and memory . . . Knowing that you *are* creating it now.   *(ample pause)*

And now . . . bringing your thoughts and creations . . . into actions . . . Remembering everything you saw and experienced . . . Breathing in oxygen, vital and energizing . . . Stretching as you need . . . Feeling open to all creativity and abundance . . . as you open your eyes to this new moment of creation.

MENTALLY CREATE YOUR DESIRE

PURPOSE: *ABUNDANCE, CREATIVITY*

SUMMARY: Connect and unite with a symbol representing abundance, creation, and expansion. Experience the feeling of having what you choose to have, or have more of, in your life.

MY EXPERIENCE: This imagery is relaxing and ethereal. Due to the longer induction, it can help analytical people relax into their imaginal minds.

EXAMPLE: Min sees a spiritual book as the symbol of his quest for spirituality. He is surprised to open the book and find a one hundred dollar bill inside. It confuses him at first, as he doesn't think of himself as materialistic or as giving money the highest priority. Then he realizes that it's a message—that having more financial abundance in the future will allow him time away from business for his esoteric studies.

ADAPTATION: You can adapt this script to just about anything: love, creativity, sobriety, mindfulness, spirituality, faith, etc. The list is endless.

STARS: INSIGHT PAGE QUESTIONS

1. What symbol did you see to represent abundance, creation, and expansion?
2. How did the symbol look as you walked around it?
3. When you joined it, how did it feel?
4. What did it mean to you?
5. What did you envision within this abundance, creation, and expansion that you want in your life?
6. How will this benefit you and those around you when you manifest this in your life?
7. What is your next step in the process?

SWIMMING WITH SEA LIFE

"Smell the sea, and feel the sky, let your soul and spirit fly." ~ Van Morrison

You're sitting on the most beautiful beach on a small crescent bay . . . at the perfect time of day . . . watching the turquoise water sparkle under the sun . . . Completely relaxed, feet in the warm, soft sand . . . You take in a breath of the fresh scent of the sea . . . with the slight smell of salt . . . Hear the soft sound of the surf . . . how the rhythmic lapping . . . disappears into silence. Palm trees rustle in the breeze . . . You are so relaxed . . . so at peace. Allowing the scents and soothing sights and sounds to lull you deeper into serenity . . . into the imagination, where everything is possible.

Now you stand up and walk into the shallow water. With your feet in the water, you feel at one with this tranquil turquoise bay. You watch the small, quiet waves lap into shore, meeting the silky white sand . . . to then recede.

You stare at the water, mesmerized . . . when suddenly you see your favorite sea life in the bay, swimming toward you! You look around to see if anyone else sees this beautiful creature. But you're alone. It's just you and this magical animal . . . as if it came just to visit you! You watch as it swims slowly in a circle and swims back, closer to you. You feel the excitement of this amazing experience! You walk farther in to submerge yourself into the water completely, and the sea animal swims toward you slowly and gracefully. And there they are, looking right at you. You feel honored and thrilled by being so close. It's as if they are asking you to swim with them. And so, you begin to swim slowly, and your new friend swims beside you. And you feel the connection in a language of movement and magical energy.

(Note: Please pause after each question to allow the participant to visualize and process.)

1. You swim a little, and float, and swim, and float again . . . alongside your special friend.
2. And now, the animal comes nearer, to look at you and allow you to touch them if you choose.
3. What does it feel like to touch the animal? And how does the animal react?
4. The animal now has a message for you.
5. You look into their eyes, and understand the message.
6. What message do they give you?
7. You have had an amazing experience . . . and it is now time to say goodbye.
8. Thank the animal for this magical time. And express whatever else you'd like to say.

Walking back into shore, you return to your place on the beach, and smile, remembering your experience. Still feeling the thrill of this chance encounter and what it meant to you. And now beginning to come back to room awareness, feeling refreshed and alert, feeling the surface under you supporting you completely, stretching, and yawning if you need to. Counting up one and two, three and four, and on the count of five, opening your eyes to the wonder of life.

BE PRESENT, CONNECT WITH SEA LIFE

PURPOSE: *BEING PRESENT*

SUMMARY: Swim with your favorite sea life. Enjoy the experience, connection, and awareness. Receive a message from the sea animal.

MY EXPERIENCE: This imagery runs from simple fun to spiritual, depending on the participant. It is simple, relaxing, and enjoyable.

EXAMPLE: Tia sees a dolphin in the bay and is thrilled. She and the dolphin swim together slowly, and the dolphin gives her the message, "We are one. We are the same, living creatures that love and feel." Tia is grateful for this beautiful experience.

ADAPTATION: You can adapt this script to a particular marine animal requested by the participant: dolphin, porpoise, sea turtle, whale, mermaid, or cartoon sea animal.

SWIMMING WITH SEA LIFE: INSIGHT PAGE QUESTIONS

1. Describe the sea animal that visited you in the bay.
2. How did you feel getting into the water with it?
3. When you joined it, how did you feel?
4. What were its qualities?
5. How did it feel swimming with it?
6. If you chose to touch it, how did it feel?
7. What message did it give to you?
8. How can you use this message in your life?

SWORD AND VASE

"Yin and Yang are one vital force—the primordial aura." ~Wang Yangming

Getting settled into the surface you're on . . . Closing your eyes . . . Taking in a long, deep breath, inhaling from your stomach, up into your chest, and releasing it as you let go of all of the day's thoughts and concerns . . . drifting down into a soothing state of serenity. Taking in another deep, deep breath . . . into the stomach . . . and exhaling anything unlike peace and serenity . . . Feeling centered, soothed, and content . . . as you rest into the stillness . . . Your body and mind drifting deeper . . . all senses soothed . . . Drifting deeper . . . into the imagination . . . to find that . . .

You're standing in an open field of green grass stretching to the horizon. You watch the grass sway from left to right and right to left in the gentle breeze. The temperature is ideal.

(Note: Please pause at each step to allow the participant time to visualize and process.)

1. As you look to the left, you notice a sword in the grass.
2. Curious, you walk to the sword and observe its shape and size.
3. Pick the sword up and feel how it feels in your hand. Feel the weight of it.
4. Look closely at it, and notice details. Observe the handle and the blade.
5. What do you think of this sword?
6. What do you like about it? . . . Or dislike?
7. And now, because we can do anything in the imagination, become the sword.
8. How do you feel as the sword?
9. What is your purpose as the sword?
10. Become yourself again.
11. You look to the right and notice a vase.
12. Walk toward it, and observe. Look at its shape, size, and color.
13. Pick the vase up. What is the weight of the vase?
14. What do you like about it? What do you dislike?
15. And now, become the vase. How do you feel as the vase?
16. And what is your purpose as the vase?
17. Become yourself again.
18. Now the sword makes a statement to the vase . . . What does it say?
19. And the vase responds. What does *it* say?
20. Thank the sword and vase for their information.

And now, beginning to return to room consciousness . . . Becoming aware of your breath . . . hearing my words and the sounds inside and outside. With each word I say . . . remembering everything you saw and experienced . . . while becoming more aware of the surface under you. Stretching your arms and legs as you take in a refreshing breath, feeling more alert . . . and gently opening your eyes, rejuvenated and revitalized . . . and ready for the rest of the day.

MASCULINITY / FEMININITY

PURPOSE: *RELATIONSHIPS*

SUMMARY: Visualize a sword and vase as you connect to the masculine and feminine aspects within you. Receive information regarding your feelings and beliefs about these attributes, intimate relationships, and your purpose within them. ***Note:*** *After receiving participant's perception of their imagery's meaning, you can look in the Universal Symbol Dictionary for further details about the sword and vase (colors, shape, texture, stones).*

MY EXPERIENCE: This imagery from Dr. Robert DeSoille (see Chapter 7, Resources) beautifully illustrates a client's feelings about masculinity/femininity, anima/animus. It's a great imagery to use when discussing intimate relationships and belief systems about one's role within a relationship.

IMAGERY EXAMPLE: Autumn sees a silver samurai sword, which she thinks is beautiful and valuable. She believes its purpose is "to fight and to protect." When she picks it up, it feels light. She enjoys wielding it in her imagination. The vase she sees is round and heavy, and she chooses not to become it. She says, "I don't know why, but it annoyed me." She said, "Its purpose is to look good, and maybe to hold flowers." She was surprised when she learned the imagery's focus. She laughed and said, "I liked the sword, and I liked the feeling of being a protector. In relationships, I know that's the role I take. My wife takes care of vases and things like that."

SWORD AND VASE INSIGHT PAGE QUESTIONS

1. Describe the sword. Where was it placed when you saw it? What was its weight?
2. What did you like about the sword? Was there anything you disliked?
3. If you became the sword, how did it feel?
4. What was the purpose of the sword?
5. Describe the vase. Where was it placed when you saw it? What was its weight?
6. How did you like it? Anything you disliked?
7. If you became the vase, how did it feel?
8. What was the purpose of the vase?
9. What did the sword say to the vase?
10. How did the vase respond?
11. How does the sword and vase's conversation relate to your intimate relationships?
12. And how can you use this to improve your relationships?

SYMBOL OF YOUR LIFE

"The symbol is greater than visible substance." ~Freya Stark

Allow yourself to get comfortable . . . Close your eyes . . . and take in a deep, relaxing breath, and release it. Feel how the surface you're on supports you completely. Take in another deep breath and release that . . . as you let go of the day. Peace and calm and calm and peace flow right and left, left and right, and right through the center. All the tiny muscles around your eyes are smooth and relaxed. All the muscles in your face, mouth, and neck relax . . . and you might even swallow in this perfect relaxation . . . as your entire body relaxes.

Let your shoulders relax into gravity, your arms . . . the palms of your hands, through your chest, heart, and lungs, down through your back and spine. Through the center . . . into your abdomen . . . down your thighs, through your knees. More and more relaxed, through your shins and calves and down into your ankles . . . into your feet. Feeling very relaxed . . . from head to toe . . . And now, imagining that . . .

(Note: Please pause at each step to allow the participant to visualize and process.)

1. In front of you, you see a symbol that represents your life at present.
2. What size is the symbol?
3. What shape and color(s)?
4. What is your overall impression of the symbol?
5. What do you like best about it?
6. What do you like least?
7. Become the symbol.
8. How do you feel?
9. As the symbol, look at you, the person. What does the person look like?
10. As the symbol, what do you want the person to know about you?
11. What advice can you give the person?
12. Become yourself again.
13. How do you feel about what the symbol said?
14. What do you want to tell the symbol?

And now, beginning to feel more aware as you come back to room consciousness. You hear my words and the sounds inside and outside of the room. You begin to stretch your arms and legs and take in a refreshing breath of air, oxygenating your body. Feeling the sensations of relaxed renewal from this journey within. Remembering what you learned as you become aware of new things, and new possibilities felt and remembered, for when it's important. Becoming more alert as you bring yourself back to room consciousness by gently opening your eyes, refreshed and rejuvenated and ready for the rest of the day.

PERCEPTION OF PRESENT LIFE

PURPOSE: *SELF-AWARENESS*

SUMMARY: See a symbol that represents your life at present and dialogue with it for better understanding. *Note: After the participant discusses the meaning of their symbol, for more qualities of the symbol (size, color, texture, etc.) look in the Universal Symbol Dictionary at the back of the book.*

MY EXPERIENCE: This is a good imagery for participants to get in touch with how they're feeling about their present life, an issue they're having, or a transition they're going through. It often surprises clients with its accuracy.

EXAMPLE: Vicki sees a beautiful blue vase that is up in the air and spinning. She loves vases but she's confused about why it's spinning in the air. When asked, "What is up in the air right now?" she replies, "I'm moving, so everything is up in the air!" The vase told her, "Let it be." She said she knows what that means. "It will all get done eventually. I just need to do what I can each day and be patient."

SYMBOL OF YOUR LIFE: INSIGHT PAGE QUESTIONS

1. Describe the symbol: its size, shape, colors, texture, and movement (if it was mobile).
2. What is your overall impression of it?
3. What did you like the most?... What did you like the least?
4. How did it feel to become the symbol?
5. When you were the symbol, what did you think of you, the person?
6. As the symbol, what did you want you, the person, to know about you?
7. What advice did you give you, the person?
8. How do you feel about the symbol, and what did you say to it?
9. How does this relate to your present life?
10. And how can you best utilize this information now?

T-SHIRT

"We are constantly invited to be who we are." ~ Henry David Thoreau

Close your eyes and become comfortable. Feel how the surface you're on supports you completely. And as I begin to count down from five to one... Counting five... feel relaxation moving down through the top of your head, through your mind, left and right and right and left. Peace and calm and calm and peace flowing from side to side and right through the center. Counting down four, relaxing more deeply with each breath you take and release. Three... more deeply relaxed with each breath... each beat of your heart... Even more relaxed to two... Deeper relaxation... So at peace... And counting way down to one... into the stillness of silence... and now, entering into the imagination... where you can go anywhere at any time. And finding that...

(Note: Please pause at each step to allow the participant time to visualize and process.)

You're walking down a city street.

1. Notice what city you're in and the activity level of the city.
2. How do you feel being here? What do you like about this city?
3. As you walk down the street, you notice that you're wearing a T-shirt . . . and that there is a symbol on the front of the T-shirt. Notice what the symbol is.
4. The people passing by might look at your T-shirt. How do they respond?
5. And how does that affect you?
6. Now you notice that there is a symbol on the back of your T-shirt. What is this symbol?
7. People walking from behind you might notice the symbol and turn around as they pass to respond. How do they respond to it?
8. And how do you react to this?
9. You see a lovely park ahead and sit down on a bench to just relax in the sun for a moment.
10. Allowing the relaxation of the sun warming you . . .

And now, beginning to return . . . Remembering everything you saw and experienced clearly . . . as I begin to count up from one to five . . . Counting up one . . . and two . . . Feeling more alert . . . relaxed and refreshed from this journey within . . . Up three and four . . . Beginning to stretch your fingers and toes . . . Feeling rejuvenated from this journey within . . . And now . . . opening your eyes on the count . . . of . . . five, to the light of the room, alert and aware and ready for the rest of the day.

WHAT YOU PRESENT AND WHAT YOU FEEL

PURPOSE: *CLARITY*

SUMMARY: Walk down a city street and notice the activity level. See a symbol on the front of your T-shirt (what you present to the world) and a symbol on the back of your T-shirt (what you feel authentically). *Note: After the participant has fully described their interpretation of their symbols, see the Universal Symbol Dictionary for further information.*

MY EXPERIENCE: This is a perfect imagery to use to introduce groups or individuals to the fun and accuracy of symbolic imagery. It's simple, short, and engaging. It can also be used as an icebreaker in newly formed groups. Though the imagery is simple, participants can get a surprising amount of information from the symbols and the city they see themselves in. The city usually relates to their interests and values and the pace at which they like to live life.

EXAMPLE: Tim sees himself in a small town where the activity level is slow. He sees a happy face on the front of his T-shirt. He says he's generally happy and friendly. On the back of his T-shirt, he sees a circle with a slash through it. He says that means, "Don't enter" or "Don't be me." He recalls that he often tells his little brother, "Don't be me; don't do what I do." He then explains that he is changing his life so that he won't be "that person that he doesn't want to be."

T-SHIRT: INSIGHT PAGE QUESTIONS

1. What city were you in, and what was the activity level?
2. How did it feel to be in this city, and what do you like about this city?
3. What was the symbol on the front of your T-shirt? Describe it.
4. What does this symbol mean to you?
5. If people noticed the symbol, how did they respond?
6. And how did that affect you?
7. Describe the symbol on the back of your T-shirt.
8. And what meaning does that symbol have for you?
9. If people noticed the symbol, how did they respond?
10. And how did that affect you?
11. How does this information relate to you at present, and how can you use it in your life?

TALK WITH THE BODY

"I learned the things you do not say tend to scream the loudest within." ~ Beau Taplin

Note: Choose an emotion, issue, or quality the participant wants to release, such as grief, fear, anger, addiction, codependency, control, procrastination, pessimism, or stubbornness.

You're sitting on the most beautiful beach at the perfect time of day ... Your feet are warm in the soft, silky sand ... You take in a breath of the misty, salted scent of the sea ... The sun sparkles off the water like diamonds. You hear the sound of the surf ... that quiet roar ... that disappears into silence ... and then returns in rhythm and rhyme. The palm trees rustle in the breeze ... You're feeling so at peace. Allowing all the scents and soothing sounds to lull you deeper into relaxation ... And into the imagination, where everything is possible.

And now, begin to get in touch with an emotion, issue, or quality you are choosing to release.

(Note: Please pause at each step to allow the participant time to visualize and process.)

1. Begin to scan your body to find where in your body this (emotion, issue, or quality) lives.
2. When you know where it is, simply place your attention on it, and send it love and acceptance, with no judgment.
3. Now, allow a symbol to appear that represents the (emotion, issue, or quality).
4. What is the symbol? *(pause)* What size is it? (pause) What color? *(pause)*
5. And what shape?
6. What are the qualities of the symbol?
7. How do you feel about it?
8. Now, give the symbol a voice.
9. Ask it what it does for you, or what it is attempting to do for you.
10. What do you want to say to it?
11. What does it need from you to do what you want it to do?
12. Tell it what you're willing to do to assist in this.
13. If the symbol is willing to change or transform, what would you like to replace it with in that part of your body?
14. If this is possible at this time, just imagine that happening now, as much as is possible.
15. Thank the symbol for appearing and giving this information to you.

Now, drawing your attention back into the present. Remembering everything you saw and experienced ... Feeling how the surface you're on supports you completely ... Breathing in a fresh breath of oxygen, vital and energizing ... Beginning to move your fingers and toes ... Stretching as you need ... Feeling light and relaxed in the present ... of the present. Comfortable in body and mind ... Flowing from the inside out ... and the outside in ... to return to room awareness ... as you open your eyes, refreshed and revitalized.

DIALOGUE WITH ISSUE THROUGH YOUR BODY

PURPOSE: *RELEASE*

SUMMARY: Connect to an emotion, issue, or quality through a symbol that you see in your body. Have a dialogue with it to get clarity on the feeling, issue, or quality that you would like to address. Discover why it is there, what it is doing for you, and how you can assist it for your benefit, in whatever way you choose.

MY EXPERIENCE: This imagery is great for kinesthetic people, who "feel" through their bodies, or have somatic symptoms. Participants can receive greater awareness of the issue with which they are dealing, and move toward transformation.

EXAMPLE: Linh sees a symbol of a chain around her ankles. She has been in a very difficult and unrewarding relationship. When she speaks with the chain, it says that it represents the fear of being alone that keeps her in her relationship. After telling the chain that she wants to leave, she says, "The chain seems relieved." The chain tells her, "I'm so tired of not being myself." When she asked the chain what she could do to help it, it said, "Let me go! We'll be happier alone."

TALK TO THE BODY: INSIGHT PAGE QUESTIONS

1. Where was the (emotion, issue, or quality) in your body?
2. What do you associate with this part of your body?
3. Do you know why the (issue) was in that part of your body?
4. What was the symbol that represented your (issue)?
5. What were the qualities of the symbol?
6. What did the symbol say it does or was attempting to do for you?
7. What did you tell the symbol about this?
8. What did it need from you to do what *you* wanted it to do?
9. Can you imagine doing this to get more of what you want?
10. If the symbol (issue) was ready to transform in any way, what did you decide you would like to replace it with in that part of your body?

TRANSFORMATION

"Change is inevitable, but transformation is by conscious choice." ~ Heather Ash Amara

Getting comfortable now . . . Closing your eyes . . . Letting all your muscles expand and relax. There is a light of the most beautiful color surrounding your entire body. Take in a breath as you inhale peace and calm from this light. Feeling and seeing the healing light all around you. Inhaling peace, and exhaling calm. Inhaling calm, exhaling peace. Absorbing its healing properties as it moves through your body, lighting up your mind, and moving down through your heart, brightening and glowing, down through your arms, into your hands . . . into your stomach, shimmering and sparkling, through your abdomen and down your legs . . . into the bottom of your feet . . . filled with the light of love.

(Note: Please pause at each step to allow the participant time to visualize and process.)

You sit outside in your favorite peaceful place in nature. Look around this familiar place and the beauty you feel so comfortable in. You are here this evening with a group of Wise Ones who have been guiding you. Some you may have met, and others you may not have. The air is pure and clean, and a few stars begin to twinkle above. There is a fire burning in the center of the circle, and you know a ceremony is about to begin. The Wise Ones look directly at you, smiling, with the light of unconditional love in their eyes. They are here to celebrate you on your present journey. They know what you have gone through—learning, growth, and even the pain. They know you are transitioning into a new time. The Wise One who stands up in the middle near the fire says the ceremony has begun.

1. The Wise One says, "We are here to *celebrate you.*"
2. All together, the Wise Ones say, "We see you, we know you. We love and honor you for exactly who you are."
3. Another Wise One stands and says, "We honor your strength," and the Wise One names your Strength. Listen.
4. And now another stands and says, "We honor your lesson." The Wise One now tells you what your Lesson is. Listen.
5. And yet another stands and says, "We give you this name, to encourage you when you need courage within." Listen to the name given to you.
6. And now, the first Wise One stands again and says, "We have a gift for you as you begin your new journey." The Wise One comes to you and hands you your gift. Notice what it is.
7. The Wise Ones now bow to you and call you by your gifted name of encouragement again.
8. The Wise One says, "We honor who you *are*, all you have *done*, and all you *will do.*"

All together they say as they look at you, "There is no more waiting. Your life is now. Live your life. Be alive *in* it." You bow to the wise ones and thank them for the ceremony and gifts.

And now, beginning to become more aware of your surroundings . . . the surface below you . . . in the outside world . . . as you prepare to come back. You might hear sounds inside or outside the room . . . and the sound of my voice . . . Becoming aware of your breathing, relaxed and regular . . . Feeling light and more alert. Taking in a breath of energizing oxygen, and bringing yourself back to room awareness, refreshed and rejuvenated, enlightened and at peace . . . as you open your eyes . . . to the light of the room.

ATTEND CEREMONY OF TRANSITION

PURPOSE: *INSPIRATION, MOTIVATION*

SUMMARY: Participate in a transformation ceremony with wise ones. Receive information on your strength, your lesson, a special name for courage, and a gift for your continued journey. *Note: Check "Quick Search" in the Universal Symbol Dictionary for information on the meaning of the landscape and gift received.*

MY EXPERIENCE: This is a meaningful imagery to celebrate the completion of a goal, a healing journey, workshop, retreat, academic graduation, rite of passage, release from prison, the hospital, or treatment.

EXAMPLE: Shauntelle sees herself in a meadow at a ceremony with female sages. She has just completed her education and is soon starting a new career. She feels great wisdom and kindness emanating from these women. They tell her that her purpose is "communicating women's strength and bringing women together for the betterment of the world." They inform her that her lesson is to learn patience, that she can't "do it all now, and it will come in time." They give her the title "Gatherer" and say that she will gather the right people at the right time to make substantial changes. They give her a compass, which she says means "confidence in choosing my direction."

TRANSFORMATION: INSIGHT PAGE QUESTIONS

1. Describe your peaceful place.
2. How did you feel in the circle with the sages?
3. What qualities did you feel from them?
4. What did they tell you your strength is?
5. What did they tell you your lesson is?
6. What special name or title did they give you for courage for your journey?
7. What does this name mean to you?
8. What gift did the Wise Ones give you for your journey?
9. How can you use this in the future?

TREE

*"But the trees seemed to know me.
They whispered among themselves and beckoned me nearer." ~ Ruskin Bond*

And now, close your eyes and let go of all the day's thoughts and concerns. Take in a deep, relaxing breath . . . deep down into your stomach . . . and up into your chest . . . Let go of anything that isn't right here and right now. Feel how the surface you're on supports you completely, allowing all the muscles in your body to relax into gravity . . . Relax deeply . . . and notice how the sounds inside and outside . . . simply add to your relaxation . . . going within . . . to the still space of silence. Enjoy this moment of complete quiet and feeling of peace . . . And now . . .

(Note: This imagery should be taken very slowly for the participant to process the experience, and the seasons. Give ample pauses at each step to allow the participant to visualize and process.)

Imagine that you are standing in front of a tree. Take a moment to closely observe it.

1. What type of tree is it?
2. Become aware of its height and its shape.
3. You can get closer and feel the energy of the tree.
4. See small details. Touch the leaves. Run your hands over the bark.
5. Walk around the tree to see it from all perspectives.
6. Observe the landscape this tree lives in.
7. Breathe in the fragrance of the earth, feeling grounded and connected to it.
8. Now, lean into the tree and imagine that you meld into it and become it.
9. How do you feel as the tree?
10. Grow roots as far down into the earth as feels natural.
11. How high into the sky do you climb? How does it feel reaching outward with your branches?
12. What are your strengths and weaknesses?
13. And what do you add to the landscape?
14. Now, experience the season of fall, when the air cools and the nights lengthen. *(longer pause)*
15. Feel the changes into winter . . . colder . . . darker . . . quieter now. *(longer pause)*
16. And into spring, when life comes alive. *(longer pause)*
17. And summer . . . warmer, longer, brighter days. *(longer pause)*
18. Now, as the tree, you receive a message of wisdom from the earth.
19. Listen and be aware of the message and the feeling it evokes.
20. Becoming yourself again, now, thank the tree for its message.

You begin to feel more alert, becoming aware of the surface under you, and sounds around you, as you begin stretching your fingers and toes. Beginning to return to the here and now . . . Remembering everything you saw and experienced clearly. Feeling safe, supported. Aware of your growth . . . Aware of your strengths . . . Open to the changes and seasons of your life . . . as you open your eyes, feeling nourished, refreshed . . . Grounded in gratitude and growth.

EXPERIENCE SELF AS TREE

PURPOSE: *BEING PRESENT*

SUMMARY: Become a tree. Feel your connection to the earth and experience the seasons as the tree. Receive a message from the earth. *Note: After fully listening to the participant's personal meaning, you can use the Universal Symbol Dictionary to look up additional qualities of the tree that was visualized.*

MY EXPERIENCE: This is a soothing, refreshing imagery to ground participants. It's also good for group work, drawing, and journaling.

EXAMPLE: Linda saw herself as a sequoia tree, which reminded her of annual gatherings at a national park her family loves. She felt strength and connection to her roots and family. She mentioned that moving through the seasons felt bittersweet to her, remembering family members who have passed. She also saw new growth in the forest, which she said represented her new career and her children's progress. The message she received from the sequoia was, "Life is eternal, family lives on."

TREE: INSIGHT PAGE QUESTIONS

1. What type of tree did you see? What was the height and shape of the tree?
2. What did you like about this tree? Was there anything you didn't like?
3. What was your overall impression of it?
4. When you became the tree, how did you feel?
5. How deep or shallow were your roots?
6. How did it feel reaching up into the sky?
7. What are the strengths of this tree? The weaknesses? And how do they relate to your strengths and weaknesses?
8. What did you, as the tree, add to the landscape?
9. How did it feel living through the season of fall? Winter? Spring? Summer?
10. What was your favorite season? And least favorite season? And why?
11. What do you and this tree have in common?
12. What message did the earth give you?
13. How can you use this message in your life?

TWO ROADS

"I am not what happened to me, I am what I choose to become." ~ Carl Jung

Get settled into the surface you're on, and close your eyes. Take in a deep, healing breath, inhaling from your stomach up into your chest, and releasing it as you let go of all of the day's thoughts and concerns . . . Drifting down into a soothing state of serenity . . . Taking in another deep, healing breath . . . into the stomach . . . Exhaling anything unlike serenity. Feeling centered, soothed and content . . . breathing in one more deep, healing breath . . . into the stomach . . . up into the chest, and releasing it . . . into stillness . . . Drifting deeper . . . into relaxation . . . all the senses soothed . . . and deeper . . . safe and sound . . . into the imagination.

You are walking up the slight incline of a small hill. You can't see over it as you continue to walk toward the summit.

(Note: Please pause at each step to allow the participant to visualize and process.)

1. You reach the summit and see two roads: one leading to the left, and one leading to the right.
2. You intuitively know that the road to the left leads to the past.
3. As you stand at the crossroads, invite a loving guide to join you on your journey to the past.
4. This person or being loves you completely and wants only the best for you. They now stand in front of you in peace and compassion. Greet your guide in whatever way you choose, feeling safe and secure in their presence.

You both begin walking down this road until you reach a place where you see a spontaneous scene from the past.

5. Let it be whatever it is, and watch it as if you're watching a movie.
6. Notice what's happening in this scene from the past.
7. What does your guide feel about this past experience?
8. Now, connect with that you from the past, and tell them whatever you need to say.
9. If you would like to comfort them, do that now, or tell them anything you'd like.
10. Now, the two of you and your guide begin walking back to the middle road. You've arrived at the road to the future now.
11. The three of you begin walking on this road to the future.
12. How does it look here, and how do you feel?
13. How does it differ from the road to the past?
14. What is happening here in the future? And how do you feel about it?
15. How does your past self feel about it? Embrace that past self, and allow them to merge into you like light, with their new perspective and information.
16. What does your guide say about the future?
17. Thank your guide in whatever way you choose now, knowing you can reconnect whenever needed.

And now, beginning to return . . . Remembering everything you saw and experienced clearly . . . as I begin to count up from one to five . . . Counting up one . . . and two . . . Feeling more alert . . . Relaxed and refreshed from this journey within . . . Up three and four . . . Beginning to stretch your fingers and toes . . . Feeling good . . . right where you are in the here and now . . . and opening your eyes on the count of five.

VISIT PAST AND FUTURE WITH GUIDE

PURPOSE: *AWARENESS, RELEASE*

SUMMARY: Walk the road to the past, watch a scene from the past, and dialogue with your past self. Receive information from your guide. Walk the road to the future, envision and experience what lies ahead, and receive information from your guide.

MY EXPERIENCE: This is a good imagery for receiving insight on the changes from the past to present and future, and normally brings hope and inspiration.

EXAMPLE: Elise met with her guide, who was a wise woman. She felt hesitant to take the road to the past. When she did, she saw herself alone and confused. She felt empathy for her past self. The wise woman said, "This isn't you anymore." Elise told her past self that life is good now and that "things get much better." She embraced her past self and asked her to come with her and the wise woman to the future. The road to the future was woodsy, with pine trees and a meadow with flowers. She saw herself there, walking with her dog and future husband, looking very happy. Elise said that she looks forward to having a partner and a family.

TWO ROADS: INSIGHT PAGE QUESTIONS

1. How did you feel as you stood at the crossroads?
2. Describe the guide that joined you on your journey.
3. How did you feel looking at the road from the past?
4. Describe the scene you saw from the past.
5. How did it feel watching it? What did you say to your past self?
6. What did your guide say about this experience?
7. And how did it feel walking down the road to the future?
8. What did you experience yourself being/doing in the future?
9. How did you feel about that?
10. And how does that relate to you at the present time?

WELCOME

*"There was a charm in being reborn into the world
when one was old enough to appreciate it." ~ Thomm Quackenbush*

Relax into the surface you're on, and close your eyes. Take in a deep, healing breath, inhaling from your stomach up into your chest, and releasing it as you let go of all of the day's thoughts and concerns . . . Drifting down into a soothing state of serenity . . . Taking in another deep, healing breath . . . into the stomach . . . exhaling anything unlike peace. Feeling centered, soothed, and content . . . breathing in one more deep, healing breath . . . into the stomach . . . up into the chest, and releasing it . . . Moving into the center of stillness . . . Drifting . . . into relaxation . . . all the senses soothed . . . and into the imagination.

You, as the adult you are today, are going back softly, safely, and gently in time, to see your mother . . . (Note: Please pause at each step to allow the participant time to visualize and process)

1. . . . in bed, holding you, as a newborn in her arms.
2. You walk to the side of the bed where your mother holds you. She looks up toward you and offers you your newborn self.
3. You gently lean over and lift Newborn You into your adult arms.
4. You feel the slight weight of your tiny body, look down into those new, innocent eyes, and send yourself love.
5. You feel how amazing and miraculous this new life is. You, this living, breathing being, new to the world. This new being is *you*, the only one of you in this world, living as you, to express as you. You know this child better than anyone ever has, or will. And you want the very *best* for them. You bring the newborn's head to your shoulder, securing them safely against your chest.
6. You feel your tiny newborn heart beating against your own and feel the newness and all the possibilities of this child. This bright, beautiful being is *you*. And you send this being *love*. As you hold the infant, you let them know that *you* are taking care of them now.
7. All their dreams, desires, joy, love, and gifts to share with the world are there inside. And you are here nourishing this precious life—*your* life. Taking care of, loving, and supporting yourself. You are aware of how special and unique this new human is . . . aware of how special and unique *you* are.
8. As you embrace this child in love and protection, you hold the back of their head, place them in front of you, and look into their shining eyes. You have an important message of wisdom to share. Tell them now . . . as you look into their eyes.
9. How does the newborn react?
10. And now you hold this precious life very close to your chest. With the light of love and wisdom, this newborn you becomes a beautiful body of pure light that merges into every cell of your body. Feel the warmth moving through every part of you, embodying this newness.
11. This spirit of newness looks out through your eyes each day. And each day as you open your eyes, you are aware of a new beginning, an amazing, miraculous new world to explore and a new being to be and become.

And now, beginning to return . . . Remembering the love and the miracle you are. Remembrances that remain . . . retained . . . Reborn in each moment . . . as I count up from one to five . . . Counting up one and two . . . relaxed, refreshed . . . up three and four. Beginning to move your fingers and toes . . . feeling revitalized and renewed . . . into the newness of each moment . . . and the miracle of you . . . and opening your eyes . . . on the count . . . of five.

CONNECT WITH NEWBORN SELF

PURPOSE: *SELF-LOVE*

SUMMARY: Connect with yourself as a newborn. Feel the essence of who you are, and the love and protection you feel for yourself. Hold your newborn self close, feeling that you are responsible to yourself and that you want to take care of yourself in the very best way possible.

MY EXPERIENCE: Many participants cry through this imagery, especially those who have been disconnected from themselves. I have also been told that this imagery is a visceral reminder that we start anew each and every day.

EXAMPLE: Cindi takes the newborn she was into her arms and holds her. She looks into her eyes and feels the love that she feels for all babies. However, she realizes that this is her. She knows what's ahead for this tiny newborn, and she tells the child, "You're going to be fine. There are good things ahead; there are challenges and pain. But there's also lots of love. You're okay, you'll do fine! And I'm here with you!"

WELCOME: INSIGHT PAGE QUESTIONS

1. What did you notice about your newborn self?
2. Describe how your Newborn Self looked.
3. How did it feel holding yourself as an infant? What did you feel *for* the infant?
4. Were there any other senses or feelings you experienced?
5. How did it feel to connect to your innocence?
6. What wisdom did you share with the newborn?
7. How can you use this information in your life now?

WELLSPRING

"Be a beneficial presence on the planet. Give your Gifts." ~ Reverend Michael Bernard Beckwith

Settle into the surface you're on, feeling completely supported. Close your eyes as you inhale peace and calm, and exhale anything unlike it. Finding yourself going deeper with each word you hear, each sound inside or outside . . . Breathing in . . . breathing out; relaxing into the silence, deeper relaxed, into inner contentment . . . journeying inward, into the imagination . . . where you find that . . .

You're walking on an earthen path through an open meadow. The ground is cool and smooth under your bare feet. Everything is vibrant and alive. A sparkling stream runs alongside your path, gently babbling over glittering rocks. Trees rustle in the breeze; their shimmering leaves reflect the sun. You hear the songs of birds—cheeps and chirps. You smell the sweet, musky aroma of the earth. The grass sways gracefully in the breeze. White clouds float through the bluest sky above you, as the sun warms your skin. Spring flowers of beautiful colors bloom as far as you can see. You breathe in their sweet fragrance, and feel a part of this continually renewing process called life.

(Note: Please pause after each step to allow the participant time to visualize and process.)

1. Up ahead, you see a wishing well. What does it look like?
2. You are curious and walk over to the well's edge.
3. As you look down into the depth of it, you see your reflection moving in the water.
4. Mesmerized, you watch its movement. Liquid light flickering your likeness below.
5. As you gaze into your depths, you know you have gifts to share with the world. And all you have to do is draw them to the surface.
6. You see a reel and a handle on the well wall. Grasp the handle, and begin turning the reel to bring your gift up. Continue reeling it up as you notice its weight. As it reaches the surface, you see it more clearly.
7. What is this gift that your wellspring supplied?
8. Now, you see a table with a chair to sit on. Place your gift on the table to observe it. Take a moment to appreciate it and understand what it means to you.
9. What do you like about your gift? *(pause)* Is there anything you don't like?
10. There might be something that helps you to share your gift with greater ease.
11. If so, let that appear in front of you now. What is it? *(pause)* And how does it assist you?

Now, thank your creative wellspring . . . Knowing it is always there within you, the ever-flowing abundance of creation . . . the stream of consciousness and creativity, always there for the taking, connected to endless possibilities and new choices in every moment.

12. Now, imagine you are sharing your gift with the world. *(pause)* What is happening?
13. How do you feel? *(pause)* And how do others respond to this gift you have shared?

Beginning to return now, grateful for this stream of infinite creation, always replenishing, always there to draw from, in the silent peace of stillness. Blessed with your own personal gifts, always new, like the stream, ever-flowing. Counting up one . . . and two . . . Feeling more alert . . . and refreshed . . . Up three and four . . . Beginning to stretch your fingers and toes . . . Feeling renewed . . . And now, on the count of five, opening your eyes to the the boundless world of possibilities.

CONNECT TO CREATIVITY

PURPOSE: *CREATIVITY*

SUMMARY: Visualize a symbol of your gift of creativity and bring it to the surface. Feel its weight and understand what it means to you. Visualize anything else that you might need to help you to manifest it, and understand the importance of sharing it with the world. *Note: After the participant has discussed their perception of their symbol, you can check the Universal Symbol Dictionary for further information on the items from the wellspring.*

MY EXPERIENCE: This imagery is a good reminder of the positives that creativity offers. It allows the participant to connect and feel what creativity means in their life. The item that helps to manifest their creativity can be anything from a person (teacher or mentor) to time, discipline, or the physical tools they use for creativity.

EXAMPLE: Rachel sees an old circular well made of brick with an A-frame roof over it. She looks into the water, reels up her gift, which is a pen. She says it represents writing. She notices that it is translucent like glass. The pen is very light, and when she picks it up, it sparkles with rainbow colors and comes alive like a holographic pen in an animated film. It begins to fly around her and create a rainbow of colors. When asked how it felt to her, she said, "Magical." When asked what is magical about writing, Rachel says, "Writing is freeing." The item she saw to help her manifest writing was a clock. She immediately said, "I've been thinking of setting up a time each day to write."

WELLSPRING: INSIGHT PAGE QUESTIONS

1. Describe the well.
2. What was your experience looking down into the water at yourself?
3. Describe the gift you brought to the surface.
4. What was its weight?
5. What does this gift mean to you?
6. Was there another item that represented something to help you manifest your creativity? If so, what was it? And how can it help you to express your creativity?
7. What do you feel your gift could mean to the world?
8. As you share your gift with others, how do you feel?
9. What do others receive from this gift? And how do they respond to it?
10. How does sharing this gift change your life and the lives of those you love?

CHAPTER 6
CONCLUSION

I hope you have enjoyed facilitating some of the 52 imageries and have experienced how valuable they can be. You have already learned some of the basics of symbolic guided imagery:

In *Chapter One* you learned that guided imagery is purposefully using the imagination utilizing the five senses, toward a goal.

In *Chapter Two* you learned the emotional, physical and spiritual benefits of guided imagery; that it can change emotional and physical states, alter a person's perspective and beliefs, and create greater awareness and inspiration.

In *Chapter Three* you learned how to facilitate the imageries: allot the time needed, prepare the environment, use your voice, and take actions if challenges arise.

In *Chapter Four* you learned the definition of symbols; the two types; personal and universal, and questions to ask the participant to better understand the meaning of their symbol(s).

In *Chapter Five* facilitating the imageries gave you the opportunity to practice and understand the power of symbolic imagery.

Remember to trust the process. The subconscious mind creates the perfect symbols to convey personal messages to participants. You need only ask questions to assist them to explore deeper meanings. Like every other skill in life, practicing imagery is the best means to become adept at it. I have listed books and organizations in Chapter 7 to guide you to further learning.

It has been my honor to share these imageries with you. I hope they bring significant discoveries and insights to you and those you work with. Enjoy exploring the ever-expansive and powerful world of the imagination!

Kathe Caldwell, CCH, GIT, CADC-II
www.hypnosissolutions.net

CHAPTER 7
RESOURCES

BOOKS ON GUIDED IMAGERY

The following recommendations include some older resources that, in part, are positively significant in innovative work in guided imagery. However, there may be parts that are outdated and/or appropriative of certain cultures. By sharing this resource list, I do not endorse any such harm to anyone or any group of people.

These are not predominantly script books but contain some scripts within them:

Assagioli, Roberto, (1965, 2000 edition). *Psychosynthesis,* The Synthesis Center.
Assagioli's classic on the nature of psychological and spiritual growth, subpersonalities, and integrating all parts of ourselves into the wholeness of being.

Beckwith, Michael Bernard, Dr., (2012). *Life Visioning,* SoundsTrue, Inc.
Self-inquiry, applying the Life Visioning process to align your knowledge and actions to your purpose.

Desoille, Robert, (1965). *The Daydream Lectures,* Sorbonne University.
Desoille's three lectures on "directed daydreaming" and its therapeutic value.

Ezra, Susan, and Terry Reed, (2008). *Guided Imagery and Beyond,* Outskirts Press, Inc.
Heartwarming personal accounts of imagery sessions, exemplifying the transformations that can be accomplished using integrative imagery.

Ferruci, Piero, (1982). *What We May Be,* Jeremy P. Tarcher.
A lovely book offering psychosynthesis techniques, written by Roberto Assagioli's protégé and collaborator.

Gottlieb, Annie, and Slobodan Pešić (1995). *The Cube . . . Keep the Secret,* HarperSanFrancisco.
The book, based on the age-old imagination game, includes interpretations and examples of celebrity outcomes.

Hay, Louise, (1984, 1990). *You Can Heal Your Life,* Hay House, Inc.
Metaphysical meanings of the body and related illnesses. Healing affirmations for body, mind, and spirit.

Jung, Carl, (1964). *Man and His Symbols*, **Dell Publishing.**

Jung's famous book on greater consciousness through interpreting symbols, metaphor, and dreams from the unconscious. Five essays by five psychologists on the unconscious, myth, individuation, and symbolism.

Leuner, Hanscarl, (1984). **Guided Affective Imagery*, **Thieme-Straiton, Inc.**

Leuner's book on mental imagery in short-term psychotherapy, used in his Guided Affective Imagery trainings.

Leviton, Charles D., and Patti Leviton, (2002) **The Conflict Between Us Is the Conflict Within Me*, **Brown Publishing Company.**

Using guided imagery and subpersonality techniques for self-awareness to improve interpersonal conflict.

Leviton, Charles D., and Patti Leviton, (2011). **The Journey Into Self*, **Trafford Publishing.**

Symbolic, therapeutic guided imagery used as a healing technique for physical and emotional issues. A great book for learning more about symbolic imagery for professionals and self-healers.

Naparstek, Belleruth, (2004). **Invisible Heroes*, **Bantam Books.**

A step-by-step program for understanding and utilizing guided imagery for PTSD, including twenty scripts.

Naparstek, Belleruth, (1994). **Staying Well with Guided Imagery*, **Hachette Book Group.**

A practical, comprehensive guide to learning the different types of imagery and how to use them for wellness. Also see heathjourneys.com, Belleruth's wonderful website, which offers hundreds of healing guided-imagery audio recordings.

Pert, Candace, (2000). *Your Body is Your Subconscious Mind,* **Sounds True.**

Neuroscientist Candace Pert, who discovered the opiate receptor, describes the powerful connection between our body/mind, consciousness, and health, from scientific observation to spirituality.

Rossman, Dr. Martin L., (2000). *Guided Imagery for Self-Healing,* **H.J. Kramer.**

A thorough resource on using imagery and the inner advisor for self-healing, by a pioneer of mind/body imagery, and one of the two original founders (with Dr. David Bresler) of the Academy for Guided Imagery.

GUIDED IMAGERY SCRIPT BOOKS

The following recommendations include some resources that, in part, are positively significant in innovative work in guided imagery. However, there may be parts of their work that are appropriative of certain cultures. By sharing this resource list, I do not endorse any such harm to anyone or any group of people.

Cedarleaf, Glenda, (2019). _A Guide for Writing and Recording Guided Imagery Meditations._
Seventy healing guided-meditation scripts are included in this comprehensive guide for writing and recording imagery.

Havens, Ronald, and Catherine Walters, (2002). _Hypnotherapy Scripts_, Brunner-Routledge.
I have included this wonderful book of Neo-Ericksonian hypnotherapy scripts as the majority of scripts are written in metaphoric prose for healing grief, depression, career challenges, medical issues, relationships, and habits.

Highstein, Max, (2016). _The Healing Waterfall_, Desert Heart Multimedia.
Over one hundred beautifully written guided-imagery scripts for counselors, healers, and clergy.

Leviton, Charles D., and Patti Leviton, (2007). _Inner Peace – Outward Power, Guided Imagery to Use With the 12 Steps to Recovery_, Aardvark Global Publishing.
Twelve imageries to use with the twelve steps of Alcoholics Anonymous; includes recordings of imageries.

Leviton, Charles D., and Patti Leviton, (2011). _The Journey Into Self_, Trafford Publishing.
Symbolic, therapeutic guided-imagery used as a healing technique for physical and emotional issues.

Lusk, Julie T., (1993). _Thirty Scripts for Relaxation Imagery & Inner Healing_, Whole Person Associates.
A compilation of scripts from different writers that include imageries for relaxation, inner answers, healing, personal growth, nature, and environment.

Schwartz, Andrew E., (1995). _Guided Imagery for Groups_, Whole Person Associates.
Offers fifty scripts for group imagery for calming, centering, creativity, congruence, clarity, coping, and connectedness.

Stapely, Louise, (2014). _Creative Visualization: 33 Guided Visualization Scripts to Create the Life of Your Dreams_.
Affirmational guided visualizations to create the life you desire.

SYMBOL INTERPRETATION RESOURCES

The following recommendations include some older resources that, in part, are positively significant in innovative work in guided imagery. However, there may be parts of their work that are outdated and appropriative of certain cultures. By sharing this resource list, I do not endorse any such harm to anyone or any group of people.

BOOKS

Andrews, Ted, (1993). _Animal Speak_, Llewellyn Publications.

The symbolism, significance, and qualities of over one hundred animals, including mammals, birds, reptiles, insects, and sea life.

Andrews, Ted, (1997). _Animal Wise_, Dragonhawk Publications.

The symbolism, significance, and qualities of more than 150 animals, including mammals, arachnids, reptiles, Insects, amphibians, fish, and sea life.

Green, Ariadne, (2001). _Ariadne's Book of Dreams_, Skylight Press.

Classic and contemporary symbols in an A-Z dictionary of dreams.

Hay, Louise, (1984, 1990). _You Can Heal Your Life_, Hay House, Inc.

Metaphysical symbolic meanings of the body and related illnesses. Healing affirmations for body, mind, and spirit.

Jung, Carl, (1964). _Man and His Symbols_, Dell Publishing.

Jung's prominent work on achieving greater consciousness through interpreting symbols, metaphor, and dreams from the unconscious.

ONLINE RESOURCES

Symbols.com

A comprehensive online symbol encyclopedia containing thousands of symbols with a helpful search feature.

IMAGERY RESOURCES

ORGANIZATIONS

Academy for Guided Imagery, Malibu, CA 90265
acadgi.com

Post-graduate training provider of Interactive Guided Imagery (IGI) for nurses, counselors, clinicians, coaches. 150-hour online program.

Association for Music and Imagery, Arlington, VA 22205
www.ami-bonnymethod.org

AMI is a nonprofit organization advancing the Bonny Method of Guided Imagery and Music (GIM). This method utilizes classical music with imagery to facilitate clients' well-being.

Imagery International, San Mateo, CA 94401
www.imageryinternational.org

International organization, raising imagery awareness. Opportunities for connection, networking, learning, and teaching. Quarterly newsletter, workshops, and annual conference.

National Center for Complementary and Integrative Health, Bethesda, MD 20892
www.nccih.nih.gov

Conducts and supports research and provides information about complementary health products and practices. Offers online CE video lectures on mind-body therapies.

ACKNOWLEDGMENTS

To my husband, Tim, who is the most loving and supportive man I have ever known. You are long on patience with me, and short on criticism. You always lean in to help. My deepest, heartfelt love and gratitude to you! You are the love of my life.

To Teri Renaud, the angel on my path who directed me toward guided imagery, hypnotherapy, and a return to the addiction treatment field. *Thank you!*

To Dr. Chuck Leviton, who first taught me symbolic imagery, and encouraged me to continue writing my own scripts. I am grateful!

Thanks to David Wessel, for kindly permitting me to use some of Chuck's imageries in this book to the reader's benefit.

Drs. David Bresler and Marty Rossman, who created the wonderful AGI program. Genius!

Thank you Katie Cross, for knowing just what to say and not to say to keep me writing.

Much gratitude to Chris Bell of Atthis Arts. He is the epitome of professionalism and wonderful to work with!

Thanks to Mothershed Designs for their work on the book cover. You made it easy.

Sincere thanks to Judy Westerfield for being a friend and mentor with the biggest, kindest heart ever.

Catherine Gardner for your amazing talent in creating the artwork for the cover of this book. You brought my vision to reality.

Thanks to Katherine Newell, Linda Newell, and Brittany Wolfe for your sterling intelligence, insight, corrections, and suggestions!

Thanks to beta readers: Pam Alexander, Dr. Vondie Lozano, and Rozanne Thompson for your time, enthusiasm, and *valuable* feedback!

Leonard Szymczak and writing group members: Thank you for your comments, corrections, and encouragement.

Kudos to my stepson, Ryan Caldwell, for your bravery through Combat PTSD to greater health and using your experience to help veterans through your program. We're very proud of you!

To Brittany Wolfe, for being my daughter from another mother. I am grateful for the fun, love, youthful enthusiasm and old soul wisdom you bring into our lives.

Thanks to friends: Diane Mead, for inspiring strength, Diane Soratos, for the wonderful memories and years of laughter, Kathryn Majewicz, for being my "Polish sister" and sounding-board in curiosity and creativity, Laura DuMaurier, for your fun, flexible, and relaxed attitude, Linda Newell for your smarts and sweetness, Pam Alexander for your vibrant, giving spirit, and . . . sassiness, Teri Renaud for your love and insight, and Vicki Canning, for your laconic wit. Each of you have enlightened my life in different ways. I'm grateful for the love and laughter you bring that helps keep me sane!

To Nickie Bethel, my affectionate and anxious childhood friend, who enjoyed being talked to sleep many-a-night by yours truly. You were unknowingly my first hypnotherapy client!

To all my cousins, for just being yourselves: fun, and loving people: Karen, Randy, Rita Marie, Penny, Paula, Tracy, Craig, April, Rob, Tia, Autumn, Mitch, Hunter, Ashly, Brook, Lauren, Kaetlyn, and Heydon.

To Lyle, who loved me completely through the first seven years of my life and helped me to know I was worthy. Your alcoholism helped me to understand from the beginning that kind, caring people can have a lousy disease.

To my father, Adolph, whose forthright intelligence inspired greater confidence in me. To my mother, Ruby, who was just the right person to raise me.

To my mother-in-law, Mary, who encouraged me to write.

Gratitude to the Fanney family: Cindi, Doug, Elise, and Ryan, for your love and support.

Love to David and Diane Dymon, who helped me to understand my family history.

To anyone I haven't mentioned who has helped in the writing of this book or helped me along my way . . . Thank You!

And thanks to all the amazing clients, students, colleagues and friends who have acted as teachers to me.

ABOUT THE AUTHOR

Kathe Caldwell currently lives in Southern California with her husband, Tim, and their comical miniature dachshund, Tobē. Like Tobē, Kathe enjoys "digging beneath the surface." She also loves the water, photography, teaching, and travel.

Twenty years ago, during the worst phase of an unexpected mystery illness, she asked for a sign and received it. It changed her career path and allowed her to live her purpose.

UNIVERSAL SYMBOL DICTIONARY

Aardvark	Time to dig beneath the surface for what you need to know. Use discernment, strength, and tenacity.
Abalone	Calming, soothing shelter.
Acacia Tree	Adaptability and endurance. Learning and resurrecting from tumultuous times.
Agate	Stability and grounding.
Air	Logic and thinking processes. Notice the condition of air: is it still, churning, windy, etc.? Air is required.
Airport	Arrivals and departures (birth/death). Newness, adventure. New ideas becoming (birth). Old ideas departing (death).
Albatross	Utilize what you have around you. Love and loyalty are important.
Allah	The God of Islam. Also known by over ninety-nine names: The Creator, The Light, The Merciful, The Most Holy, etc.
Alligator	Alligators are excellent mothers, representing new birth and creation. They thrive in mud, the mixture of earth and water that nourishes growth. Their eyes, high on their heads to see above water, remind us of "higher vision." They also digest very slowly, reminding us to "take in new knowledge slowly as to digest it."
Aluminum	Recycle old belongings and beliefs and open space for the new.
Amber	Going within for ancient wisdom and healing. Warmth and empowerment.
Amethyst	Peace, beauty, and healing of wounds through intuition and spirituality. Prayer and protection.
Anchor	A steadfast foundation is required, unless it is too weighty for you.
Angel	Protection, guidance, and spiritual assistance for you and your desired goal.
Ankh	Ancient Egyptian symbol of eternal life, wisdom, health, and prosperity. Within the ankh is the oval (birth/creation), as well as the signs of woman and man creating life.
Ankles	How can you be more flexible to move forward at present?
Ant	Ants work hard and as a team. This is the time to use the support of a team while working toward your goals.
Anteater	Trusting your own pace and intuition will assist you.

Antelope	Antelopes are capable of great speed. They are highly attuned to the environment around them and quickly adapt. A reminder that you can replenish yourself in your present environment and make quick use of your resources and ideas to create what you need.
Antlers	Protection through spirituality and regeneration of the spirit.
Ape	There is a need for clear, precise communication. Be aware of balancing strength and gentleness.
Apple	Knowledge of the duality of life, health, happiness, and longevity. Love of family and generosity.
Apple Blossom	Hope, lightness, inspiration.
Apple Tree	Wanting love and affection. Family life and generosity important.
Aquamarine	Peace, tranquility, balance. Truth in communication and emotions.
Arguing	Are you arguing against your self or others?
Archangel Gabriel	Revealer of visions.
Arms	Are you feeling able to hold all of life's experiences now? Open up, express, and connect with others.
Armadillo	Notice that sensitivity is sometimes hidden under tough exteriors. There is strength in vulnerability with discernment.
Arrow	Notice which way arrow is pointed. Up = optimism, spirituality; Down = feeling down, in mood or behavior; Left = past or left behind; Right = future. Look at N,S,E,W.
Ash Tree	Strong, ambitious. Needing to be functional, useful, and needed. Use your talents and praise others to be praised yourself.
Aspen Tree	Transformation and strength through community, communication, and cooperation.
Asphalt	Needing a strong foundation for the journey ahead.
Attic	Higher mind, things left behind or incomplete (items from childhood, etc.). Observe any items you see in the attic and determine what they represent.
Avalanche	Strong emotions that need to be released. Also signifies feeling overwhelmed by life stresses. Expression of feelings and lessening of pressure is needed.
Baboon	Stay grounded and maintain a safe space for you and your loved ones. Family and loved ones are sacred, as are work and creative efforts. Love and protect them.
Baby	New ideals awakening within you. Giving birth to something new in your life. Consider the condition of the baby and its temperament. Is it healthy, happy, etc.?
Back	Support (emotional or financial) or lack of it. Higher back= feeling weighed down by life; Mid-back=leftover issues from the past; Lower back=issues of financial support.
Back Door	Not in the open. Something that is unknown by most, hidden, or not discussed.
Badger	Self-expression, storytelling, digging beneath the surface, developing self-reliance.

Balloon	Childhood, simplicity, freedom. Celebration, or letting go. What is happening with the balloon? Are you holding on to it, or letting it go and watching it move up into the air?
Banyan Tree	Groundedness, endurance. Stay grounded and create positive boundaries with others now.
Barn	Animal instincts. Feeling open and vulnerable to living with others and their habits.
Baobab Tree	Survivor. Being positive and using the resources you have at hand allows you to thrive.
Barracuda	Pull away from the group; better to go it alone. Do not call unneeded attention to yourself or try to impress.
Basement	Subconscious mind, primal needs and desires. Can also represent those things you prefer not to deal with, the lower sphere of life and life's choices. Explore the condition of the basement for more understanding.
Bass	Balance between male and female qualities. You have many activities going at once; be as fertile as possible and a percentage of those activities will bring forth fruit.
Bat	Transition, rebirth from within. Releasing old fears. Promise of a new beginning.
Bathing	Cleansing the mind, body, spirit of old beliefs. Refreshing, renewing.
Bathroom	Cleansing and releasing. Mind, body, spirit. Consider the condition of bathroom for more understanding.
Beach	Where land (foundation/groundedness) and sea (subconscious/emotions) meet. A message to find balance and groundedness in your emotions. The need for relaxation, rejuvenation through nature.
Bear	Going within to awaken inner resources to begin using for betterment in your life. Meditation is beneficial.
Beaver	Planning, building for the future.
Bedroom	Your private life and time. Rejuvenation, intimacy, and sex.
Bee	Work, plans, group support, and activity. Creating in an organized manner. Enjoying the sweetness and beauty of your success.
Beech Tree	Needing depth, culture, and physical activity.
Beetle	The beetle has hardened forewings which protect its delicate hindwings. They are a quarter of all the described species on earth, which speaks to protection and survival through adaptation.
Begonia Flower	Storing beauty and energy within for the right time to blossom.
Bell	Bringing attention. What is it the bell brings your attention to?
Bicycle	Balance needed to move forward in life. Notice the environment and how you see and experience the bicycle.
Birch Tree	Love of nature and calm environment. Healing qualities. Need to share feelings.
Bird	Transcendence. Intuition. Spirit/soul. Rising above on one's spiritual journey. Study the type of bird you see and its qualities.

Birth	Upcoming birth. Birth to higher self, creative endeavor, or new ideas/values.
Black	Mystery, hidden, unknown. Death/rebirth, transformation through introspection.
Black Widow	Weaving the dreams today that you want to fulfill tomorrow. Be direct and straightforward. Trust the subtle messages you receive. It is time to use your creative talents to fulfill your potential.
Blackbird	Pay attention to nature and your surroundings.
Blood	Circulation of life. Can also refer to relatives or relationships.
Blue	Expression, voicing the authentic self, "true blue," peace, tranquility. Sad: "feeling blue."
Blue Jay	Developing your innate talents and proper use of power. Keep balance of work and pleasure.
Blue Tang Fish	The color blue relates to communicating your true feelings and expressing your authentic self. The blue tang has a strong tail (balance), reminding us to find balance within our daily activities and relationships.
Blue-green	Using the power of spiritual principles to bring strength to others.
Bluebird	Joy, gentleness, unassuming confidence. Connecting with authentic self and feeling the joy of self-worth.
Boat	How you deal with and express your emotions. Is the boat on calm or turbulent waters? Is the water clear or murky?
Bobcat	Learning to be alone without loneliness. Comfort in silence. Do not become overwhelmed by your environment. Trust your instincts.
Body	Your vehicle in this world. Note its condition, what stands out about your body, and how you feel about it.
Bones	Your beliefs, i.e. "down to the bone."
Box	Open box = prospects. What do you choose to fill it with? Or, feeling "boxed in." Note qualities of the box seen.
Boy	Youthful, idealistic, active male aspects. "Doingness."
Breast	Feminine, nourishing, giving, mothering.
Breath	The ability to take in life and live fully.
Brick	Solid, strong, unyielding. In what structure is the brick used? See house, wall, etc. for further understanding of the brick's purpose.
Bridge	Transition from one time or situation to another.
Brown	Earth, foundation. Growth through stability, earnestness, hard work, practicality.
Buddha	Enlightenment, compassion, generosity, patience. Buddha defined: One who is awake.
Buffalo/Bison	Abundance through staying grounded and following the easiest path. Don't make it harder than it is.

Building	What is the building used for? Grocery store = food/home needs; Library = stimulating the mind, learning; Police = protection/authority; Theater = entertainment
Bull	Power, determination, fertility. Stability without stubbornness. Envelop the feminine energies within yourself.
Bus	Traveling with others (public transportation). Notice the size, condition of the bus, and how many others are with you. Indicates how you are moving forward on your journey within a community.
Butterfly	Transformation: acknowledge and accept the changes occurring. You are stronger than you think. Look forward to authenticity, joy, and lightness.
Camel	Endurance, adaptability. Though your journey might feel difficult, with positivity and determination you can accomplish anything.
Camellia Flower	Love, affection, admiration. Longing for union.
Canary	Awakening your own voice. Healing and enlightening others and yourself through expressing your own feelings.
Car	Represents the self and aspects of self. Examine the qualities of the car: color, interior, exterior, as well as the feeling the car elicits.
Carbon Fiber	Know that great strength and flexibility can coexist; malleability is important.
Cardinal	Renewed vitality, knowing your importance.
Carnation	Love, luck, and longevity.
Carp	Patience needed for making progress. Continue forward and use all opportunities.
Cat	Self-direction, self-approval, and independence. Going inward, focusing on yourself to attain greater independence through learning positive new survival skills.
Caterpillar	Patience, hard-work, and evolution. Know that all of your endeavors will come to fruition.
Catfish	Use discernment when you speak, protect the words you say, and write. Use words carefully, for the good, and they will work for you, not against you.
Cave / Cavern	Deeper, lower levels of the mind. The shadow aspects of self that we sometimes resist and ignore.
Cedar Tree	Strength, endurance. Healing, purifying and fragrant. Used in spiritual prayer.
Centipede	New psychic connections. Pay attention to your dreams: they can provide insight and support to you. Create a positive environment for yourself to re-energize.
Chameleon	Be patient and adapt to your environment. Make your decision after weighing all options. When secure, embrace your opportunity with full commitment.
Chased, Fleeing	Being chased by your own creations. What are you feeling fearful of?
Check Sign	Accomplished, accounted for, correct.
Cheetah	Act swiftly now to succeed; give it your all. Protect your environment and those you love. Attend to your hurts and others'.

Cherry Tree	Beauty and impermanence. Reminds us that life is beautiful, yet fragile. Appreciate the love and beauty all around you, as it is always in change. Feel safe within the change.
Chest	Our feelings of love and fear. Intimate relationships.
Chestnut Tree	You have healing qualities. Balance of feminine (yin) and masculine (yang) qualities. Bring your desires into the outer world and act on them to succeed. A reminder to eat a more natural diet.
Chickadee	Innocence of childhood, joy, and playfulness.
Chicken	Fertility, sexuality, and sacrifice. Reminder that you have the power of choice in whom you give to.
Chimpanzee	It is time to be social and use the tools available. Reflect on your life and use the opportunities given you.
Chipmunk	You have a natural curiosity about life. Slow down, listen. Examine your life and plan ahead.
Christian Cross	Christ, God, spirituality, love. Representing Christian values and beliefs.
Chrysanthemum	Optimism, strength, and a joyful heart.
Circle	Wholeness, inclusion, completion, balance of power, belonging, embracing.
Circle (dot in center)	Home, self.
Citrine	Strength, attracting financial abundance, and success.
City	Community, variety, flexibility, and adaptability. Notice the qualities of the city: what the city is known for, and its meaning for you.
Clam	A message to stay open and truthful in relationships. Examine your part in being open or closed to intimacy.
Clay	Clay can be "formed." What do you choose to reform yourself into? Note the context of clay within your vision.
Cliff	Where are you in relationship to the edge of the cliff? Are you feeling unsafe or in danger? Change needed.
Clock	Time. Study numbers you see on the clock for more information. If clock is "racing," this represents that you feel you don't have enough time.
Clothing	The type of clothing you have on represents what you present to the world and activities in your life. Is clothing formal, casual, or for work? Is it appropriate to the activity seen?
Cloud	Between the seen and unseen. Manifesting your thoughts into reality. If the cloud is blocking out light, can mean "clouded thinking" or feeling sadness.
Cobalt	You are a survivor; capable of going through tumultuous times, retaining your hope and individuality.
Cobra	If you are not sure how to react now, do not react at all. Do not let others distract you. Trust what you feel despite outside appearances. Wait until you are certain.

Cockatoo	It is time to question a relationship. Is one person doing too much? Strengthen relationship through mutual responsibility.
Cockroach	Adaptability and using available resources. Messenger of cleanliness and cleansing.
Concrete	Strong and unyielding to the positive or negative in your life. Are you being too strong and unyielding, or do you need more strength? Consider how the concrete is used in your dream or imagery.
Condor	Linking the physical world with the spiritual in powerful ways to rise above previous limitations.
Copper	Earthy, supportive, protective, and nurturing. Energy conductor. Are you balanced in giving and receiving? Are you needing more energy?
Cougar	Coming into your own power and asserting with gentleness. Take charge of your life.
Cow	Nourishment, motherhood. Greater self-esteem through self-reflection and self-knowledge.
Coyote	Balancing fun and wisdom for your best life. Need for mental stimulation and close family ties.
Crab	Protection and defense. Do you feel you have to isolate? Consider sensitivity and reclusiveness. It is time to come out of your shell now.
Crane	Focus on what's truly important to you now and give it all your attention. Keep your creativity and dreams alive through action.
Cricket	You can rely on your dreams and heightened sensitivity. Trust in what you have always believed. Your beliefs will be rewarded.
Crocodile	Primal strength. It is time to bring your feelings to the surface for release. Trust your instincts now, take advantage of opportunities. Be mindful of your words.
Cross	Christian cross= Jesus, Christian beliefs. A simple cross (4 equal sized arms)= A meeting point, decisions, at a crossroad.
Crossing Bridge	Going through a time of transition. Crossing over from the seen to the unseen world or from one circumstance to another.
Crow	Create and manifest the magic of life in your everyday life. Intelligence and adaptability. Others will see your deeds; there is no need to call them to others' attention.
Cruise Ship	Desiring to cruise through present life issues, having others support and take care of you. Wishing for relaxation and replenishment.
Crucifix	Represents sacrifice; specifically of Jesus Christ on the cross and the Christian belief that his death and crucifixion redeemed humankind.
Crying	Releasing tears of joy or sadness. Do you need to express your feelings?
Crystal	Pure, transparent, spiritual, magical.
Cuckoo	Listen to and follow your intuition. Eliminate the negative. New fate.
Cypress Tree	Strong, sensitive, and empathetic. Healing qualities. Capable of dealing with others' emotions well. Reminder to not get bogged down by others' feelings.

Daddy Longlegs	Can indicate a loss of balance in a relationship. Gentleness is true strength. Communication creates greater understanding. Discuss obstacles to move beyond them.
Daffodil	Hope, rebirth, new beginnings.
Dahlia	Inner strength, change, dignity. Lasting bond between two people.
Daisy	Innocence, purity, and joy.
Dam	Holding in, holding back emotions.
Dark Blue	Intelligence, knowledge, sincerity, integrity.
Death	Death of old ideas, attitudes, beliefs, or relationships. Death is transition of the old, to allow the new to develop.
Deer	Gentleness, innocence, spirituality. Use your senses to understand subtle messages around you. Express gentle love to yourself and others. Forgive yourself.
Demon	Disowned part of self; the shadow with its own desires and primal needs.
Desert	Adaptability, using available resources, moving through challenges, purification.
Diamond (shape)	Clarity, wisdom, possibilities.
Diamond (gem)	Clarity and wholeness. A diamond ring indicates relationships, love, and commitment. Consider aspects of the diamond (color, shape, etc.)
Dining Room	How you nurture others.
Dinosaur	What is primitive, ancient, extinct, or out-of-date in your life?
Dog	Loyalty, unconditional love, companionship. Note the qualities of the individual breed of dog.
Dolphin	Fun, sexuality, energy. Sound and breath healing encouraged. Breathe new fun, activities, and spirituality into your life.
Donkey	Awakening wisdom; service and humility. Release stubbornness and complacency.
Door	Transition. Is door open or closed? If opening, new start. If closing, saying goodbye to the old.
Dove	Peace, creativity, feminine energy. Mourn the old, and look with hope to the new. Believe in the love, abundance, and magic available in the world.
Dragon	Mythical messenger of strength, courage, and power.
Dragonfly	Attune to the lightness and joy of creativity and change.
Drift	Losing bearings, emotionally and spiritually. Unsure, feeling alone.
Duck	Ducks live on land and water. A message to handle emotions and stay grounded. Emotional comfort and protection. Self-nurturing.
Dust	The most subtle matter in the universe, between matter and spirit. Is the dust magical and mystical, or simply something you sweep under the rug?
Dying	A change in consciousness; old self or old ways dying. Also, a message to de-stress.

Eagle	Eagles have amazing vision and the ability to see long distances. They are persistent and purposeful toward their goal.
Ear	Hearing what is being said.
Earth	Mother Earth. Wholeness and inclusion of the natural world and all in it. Your own body, your spiritual home. Trusting that you have all you need.
Earthquake	Feeling "ungrounded" and unsafe in life, as if your foundation is falling beneath you.
East	Moving toward the future. Goals. New beginnings.
Eating	Examine type of food you were eating. Possibly a change in diet suggested.
Eel	There is a great spiritual journey ahead, of depth and distance. You will grow stronger and be physically and spiritually transformed.
Egret	Grace, elegance, and purity. Awakening of new passions.
Eight	Creating abundance through confidently using the gifts you were given. Balancing work with spiritual principles to support self and others.
Elbow	Accepting changes and new experiences.
Elephant	Ancient wisdom and power. Spirituality, kindness, and affection. Caring for the young, elderly, and sick.
Elevator	Indicates spiritual elevation. Are you traveling up or down in the elevator? Up=going toward the higher self; Down= going toward the shadow self.
Eleven	Double strength of number 1: new beginnings, duality, balance between masculine and feminine energy. A reminder to be present. Attune to the higher vibrational energy available to you. Doorway between the physical and metaphysical.
Elk	Strength, power, stamina, and protection. Need for companionship and group support. Diet affecting energy and strength.
Elm Tree	Are you being tough on yourself or others? Release superficial concerns, and focus on a deeper connection with yourself.
Emerald	Healing and balancing the heart. Growth, rest, and rejuvenation.
Eucalyptus Tree	Strength, survival, healing, and protection.
Eyes	What we see and understand.
Face	What we show to the world. Also, a metaphor for "facing" something. Examine details of the face you see.
Fairy	Magical, nurturing spirits of guidance and light.
Falcon	You might feel like your progress is slow, but you can accelerate your efforts. Allow the sacred gift within your life to come to light.
Famous Person	What does this person represent to you? Notice the first thoughts you have about this person.
Feathers	A reminder of lightness, beauty, love, and spirituality. You can choose to rise above.

Feet	Represent our ability to move forward in life.
Fiberglass	Represents reinforcement and insulation.
Fig Tree	Are you feeling vulnerable and exposed? Use this time as a growth period in which to open up and communicate, creating greater peace.
Finch	More activity and increased opportunities. New people from diverse backgrounds in your life.
Fingers	Indicate the details of life and how we deal with them. Thumb= intellect and worry; Index= ego and fear; Middle= anger and sexuality; Ring=unions and grief; Little= family and pretending.
Fire	Passion, releasing/purification, creativity.
Firefly	A hopeful time to realize dreams. Let your light shine and get your creative ideas out into the world. Spiritual gifts are alight. Inspiration and great reward.
Fishing	Seeking spiritual self and serenity.
Five	Represents activity and manifestation. Change, in whatever activity with which it is associated.
Flamingo	Flirtation. Lessons of the heart. Discernment in love and expression of true feelings.
Flea	Until changes are made, the irritations you experience will continue.
Fleur-de-lis	The fleur-de-lis is a stylized lily, which originated in France and was used as an emblem for royalty. It came to represent purity and spirituality in feminine form. It has been used as a symbol of the Holy Trinity and is also known to exemplify faith, wisdom, and chivalry.
Flower	Blossoming potential, brightness, happiness, and new beginnings.
Fly	Remain stable through unhealthy experiences and environments. They will pass.
Flying	Rising above your challenge. Connecting with higher faculties, spiritual essence. Desiring freedom.
Fog	Confusion, fear, lack of clarity. Inability to see, understand. Wait until you can see clearly before making a decision.
Forest	Growth free of constrictions, connecting with the natural world and feminine forces, the unconscious mind.
Fork in Road	Choice between two disparate things: healthy/unhealthy, love/fear, past/future.
Forty	A period of testing and tribulation, the number is mentioned over one hundred times in the Bible.
Fountain	Flowing water, spirituality, rejuvenation.
Four	Symbolizes man in physical form in the material world. Four also represents the four corners of the earth (north, south, east and west), as well as the fours elements (earth, water, air and fire). A foundation.

Fox	Stay focused on your creative energy. Feminine forces. You can hear what isn't being said; tune in and blend with your surroundings for great wisdom.
Frog	Coming into your own creative power, learning how to control emotions and the words you choose to share. Living in water (emotions) and being grounded (earth).
Fur	Protection and warmth. Notice the condition of the fur which relates to protection. Is it healthy or unhealthy?
Garden	Controlled growth, creativity, and nourishing self and life.
Gardenia	Refinement, elegance. Often used for weddings because of their simplicity and sweet fragrance.
Garnet	Stone of strength, healing, and spiritual regeneration.
Gecko	If you are feeling opposition around you, restore order or conflicts through action as quickly as possible.
Gila Monster	Gila monsters can live two to three years without a meal. This is a message to realize that you have what you need. Maintain the resources you have, protect yourself, and believe in your abilities.
Girl	Youthful, sensitive female aspects of self. "Beingness."
Genitals	Male and female aspects of self as well as sexuality, or feeling shame within sexuality.
Giraffe	Seeing the big picture, looking ahead, being prepared. Neck = communication. Important to communicate your feelings now. Also can be a message to utilize both your heart and head.
Gladiola	Strength and passion.
Glass	Transparency, strength, and vulnerability. Glass is strong, yet vulnerable, in that it can be broken. Broken glass can represent a shattering of old beliefs and identity, i.e. your view of life at present.
Goat	Important to stay grounded and balanced on your journey toward your goals. Plan carefully to move to new heights.
God	The Creator. Creative force and energy. The Alpha and Omega.
Goddess	The universal divine feminine, expressing intuition, creation, wisdom, magic, mystery, and psychic insight. Embodied as mother, maiden, crone.
Gold (color)	Prosperity, what we "treasure," prominence, authority, grandeur, extravagance.
Gold (metal)	Illuminating the path to success. Pay attention to what you treasure. Gold also represents prosperity, wealth, authority, and glamour.
Goldfish	Desiring peace and prosperity. Use your intuition in business and work. Create a sacred and peaceful place for yourself to relax.
Goose	Symbol of 8: infinity, fertility, fidelity.
Grapes	Abundance, prosperity, fertility, pleasure, and joy. A symbol of the many gifts of God to humankind.

Granite	Strength, endurance, beauty, diversity.
Grasshopper	New leaps forward. Trust your instincts. Focus on the new. Grasshoppers only leap up or forward.
Gray	Mind (gray matter). Balance between black-and-white/all-or-nothing thinking. Intelligence, wisdom, and maturity.
Green	Healing, growth, nature, fertility. Heart, compassion, and hope. Ecology.
Groundhog	Going deep into your life interests. Explore the mysteries of death, dying, and rebirth.
Grouse	Expression and release through movement and rhythm is beneficial at this time.
Guinea Pig	Seek out groups for healing work. Spend time with people who are like-minded.
Hail	A feeling of adversity and punishment. Is self-forgiveness needed?
Hair	Our connection to the metaphysical, spiritual world and our thoughts that create physical manifestations.
Hallways	A place of transition, change.
Hamsa	An ancient middle eastern symbol of a hand with an eye within, representing protection, happiness, good luck and fertility.
Hands	Ability to share ourselves and our gifts in life. To hold and to handle life and those we love.
Happy Face	Happiness, friendliness, or projecting happiness.
Hat	Your thoughts and attitudes toward life.
Hawk	Childhood visions and dreams being realized toward your life purpose. Be open to new ideas and inspiration.
Hazelnut Tree	Groundedness. You create a nurturing environment for others. Love and companionship are very important to you, as well as wanting to feel needed.
Head	Consciousness, intellect, ego. Creation through our thoughts. Connection to the divine.
Heart	Love, relationships, self-love, and security.
Heart Chakra	The fourth chakra (anahata): related to the heart being balanced, open, pure, expansive. Color: green.
Hedgehog	You might feel the need to protect yourself. Use this time to feed your curiosity, and share your insights as you learn.
Heron	Time to balance your life using your curiosity, self-determination, and persistence. You appreciate grace and nobility.
Hibiscus	Exotic beauty and charm.
Hips	Carry us forward with good balance.
Hippopotamus	Examine and utilize your own artistic and healing powers.
Horse	Heightened sensitivity. Time to awaken to your own power and freedom. Movement is important to de-stress.

Hotel	A place of temporary housing. Relaxation or luxury. Explore the feeling you have about this hotel and its environment. What feels temporary at this time in your life?
House	Self, and aspects of the self (rooms of the house). Study specific rooms of the house that are applicable.
Hummingbird	Finding joy in your life. Believe in miracles and know you can surpass your challenges.
Hyena	Trust your own perceptions. Your ability to discern and decide is strengthening. Take yourself seriously.
Ibis	Sacred bird of ancient Egypt. It ate even poisonous snakes (transformation). Thus, the ibis is considered a bird of great healing and magic.
Ice	Frozen feelings that need to be "thawed" and expressed.
Ice Skating	Moving through your life ignoring feelings that you push underneath. Notice how you feel as you skate: feeling safe, or "skating on thin ice."
Iguana	Time to release those things no longer beneficial to you. Let go and work on new goals instead of repeating past mistakes.
Infinity Sign	Represents the infinite universe and infinite everlasting time. All that was, is, and will be: Alpha to Omega.
Intestines	Assimilation and absorption for energy.
Iris	Unique. Faith, hope, and wisdom.
Iron	Abundance, masculine energy. Power, growth, protection.
Ivy	Strong emotional attachments are a factor. Healthy boundaries important.
Jaguar	Reclaim your power and become a master over your instincts. Be patient and don't let the past stop you from accomplishing in the present.
Jasmine	Love, beauty, sensuality, and purity. Healing through scents.
Jaw	The words you say to others. Notice how you are expressing yourself.
Jellyfish	By reorganizing, you will succeed. If you are trying to do it alone, begin asking for help and divide work into smaller tasks.
Jesus	The Christ, the central figure in Christianity. The son of God, teacher of peace and forgiveness.
Jet	Power, speed, and motion. Gaining direction and authority.
Jungle	Confusion. Emotional, physical and/or financial survival issues.
Kangaroo	Experience is the best teacher. Disconnect from the past and mature. Progress with balance and stamina. Keep moving forward.
Kidneys	The kidneys are our filter, filtering out what is unneeded to purify our blood, allowing life. What needs to be released in your life?
Kitchen	How you nurture yourself. What is in the cupboards and refrigerator? What is the condition of the room?

Koala	You are stronger than you know. Your sensitivity and individuality require time alone to cleanse and heal.
Koi Fish	Determination and perseverance leading to success. Do not give up. Adapt to your present environment; you will thrive as you practice flexibility.
Kookaburra	Healing through closing the doors to the past and welcoming the future. Embrace the joy of family, friendship, and laughter. Look at the brighter side of life.
Ladybug	You do not need to push too hard for dreams to come true. Allow your desires to manifest in their own time.
Lagoon	Stillness, shelter. Look at activity/emotions below the surface.
Lake	Emotions. Contained, receptive, and wise. Feminine energies of absorption, inner power, and passivity. Note conditions of the water: is it still or disturbed?
Landslide	Feeling extreme emotions that need to be released. Feeling that your life is not stable at present.
Lapis Lazuli	Connecting with higher power, wisdom, spirituality to communicate into the world.
Lark	The lark is one of the few birds that sings while it is flying. A reminder to stay cheerful through your endeavors.
Laughing	Focus more on the lighter side of life. Seek and experience joy.
Laurel Tree	Nobility, victory, truth, and honor. Self-moderation and balance.
Lava	Have you felt long-standing anger, frustration, or resentments that you need to release? Find proper channels to express and forgive. If lava has cooled, so has your anger. If you walk on lava, that represents the ability to tolerate or endure others' anger and frustration.
Lavender (color)	Femininity, grace, tenderness, calm elegance, higher power/purpose.
Lavender (flower)	Serenity, healing, relaxation. Soothing, sleep for rejuvenation. Good for neurological challenges.
Laying Down	Relaxed, needing to regain energy, or "laying down on the job."
Lead	Toxic metal representing death and transformation. Time to cleanse impurities and imperfections from within.
Leech	Detoxification and purification. Allow yourself to feel joy, vitality, and energy.
Left	Can represent the past, "left behind" or left brain functions: analytical, practical, detail-oriented.
Left Side of Body	Represents mother, femininity, receiving side, taking in.
Legs	The power and strength to move us forward. Are you ready and prepared to move forward? Is there anything else you need?
Lemon Tree	Cleansing, purification, and stimulation. It is time to cleanse the mind, body, and spirit of negative emotions. Renewal and rebirth.
Lemur	Highly sensitive to what is not seen and not heard. Your psychic ability is increasing.

Leopard	The strength and vitality you need is available to overcome old patterns that hold you back. Giant leaps are possible.
Library	Study, learning/lessons, desire for knowledge, wisdom, research.
Lightning	Electricity, shock, excitement, surprise.
Lilac	Hope, innocent love, renewal.
Lily	Humility and the soul's rebirth.
Lime Tree	Warm, exotic climates for health. Adaptability and ability to turn negative situations into positive. A healthy diet to de-stress.
Lines	Linear= ideas manifesting into matter. Boundaries, thoughts.
Lion	Strength, courage and protection. Lions are powerful but choose not to fight uselessly. They roar as a warning; a message to use your voice for assertion, not aggression. The lion's mane is a symbol of health and power. Masculine energy reminds you to take action for your betterment.
Lioness	The lioness is a powerful protector of her cubs and provides for them by hunting. A message to honor your feminine energy: intuition, creativity and nurturing nature. A reminder to use your power assertively, not aggressively.
Lips	Secure and worthy in speaking up for one's self.
Liver	Releasing the toxic experiences of life.
Living Room	Represents your life and daily activities.
Lizard	Subtle perceptions, becoming more conscious through dreams and intuition.
Llama	Stay grounded. Climb slowly and securely to your goals with clarity.
Lobster	Are you carrying the past with you as protection? It is time to regenerate and decide how much protection is needed. Lobsters "molt" and release their shells and then regrow them. A cycle of regeneration is ensuing.
Locking Door	Wanting to lock out unpleasant experiences or thoughts.
Loon	Melancholy, imagination, bringing dreams alive.
Losing Valuables	Losing sight of what's important. Slow down, be grateful for, and watchful over valuables.
Lotus Flower	Preciousness of life, ever-unfolding. Patience to trust life and self to develop naturally.
Lungs	Ability to breath in life fully.
Lynx	Learning spiritual lessons and knowledge. Intuition is high. Seeing the unseen and hearing the unsaid.
Macaw	Sunshine, healing through time in the outdoors. Learning by repetition and expression of spiritual learnings and healing.
Magnolia Tree	Beauty, endurance, sweetness of life. Creating beauty from your interior life (yin) and sharing it with the world.

Manatee	Slow down to feel your emotions and release them. Take the slow and steady route. Open up to others and allow your vulnerability.
Mango Tree	Prosperity, fertility, and variety. Mangoes are also very healthy, their leaves having antioxidant and antimicrobial properties.
Maple Tree	Independent, distinctive, original. Needs variety and is sometimes the center of attention. Able to bring lightness and joy into situations. Hard working, functional, and nurturing.
Marble	Grounding, clarity, self-mastery, stability.
Marshes	Letting go of past emotions and stages of life. Starting anew.
Meadow	Nourishment, abundance, fertility, and growth. Safety, serenity.
Meadowlark	The meadowlark is actually a blackbird. Indicates cheerfulness, joy, and self-discovery.
Meerkat	Solidify relationships within your community. Maintain energy and fun.
Mercury	Toxic metal, representing death, mystery, and transformation. Movement, change, fluidity.
Metal	Strength, fortitude, tenacity.
Mirror	Looking at yourself. Reflection of self.
Mockingbird	Finding your purpose; recognizing your innate talents and expressing them.
Mongoose	Defense, protection, and courage. Let go of negative people, environments, and emotions and focus on your needs.
Monkey	Group socialization is important now. Express yourself clearly and ask questions. Enjoy learning and teaching through communication.
Moon	Feminine energies, yin. Passive, soothing, reflective light.
Moose	Maternal forces, survival, and protection. Pay attention to your inner world for greater strength and awareness.
Mosquito	Are you feeling irritated and attacked by others? Take care of unresolved issues to get back to center to increase self-worth and confidence.
Moth	A time for greater physical sensitivity, trusting your own senses. Awareness in intimate relationships.
Motorcycle	Suggests a need for adventure and freedom from life stressors. Note details of motorcycle and in what context it is seen.
Mountain	Overcoming obstacles, determination, and spiritual growth. Communion with higher power. Yang energy to attain goals.
Mouse	Focus and pay attention to details to attain your dreams. Take care of the small things to attain the bigger things.
Mouth	The nourishment and new experiences you take in, and the words you express to others.

Mule	Mules are unique, aware, and intelligent. They were used for transportation in Ancient Egypt (pre-camel) for their endurance, strength and sure-footedness. They can be less reactive than horses; a message to stay emotionally and physically grounded and stay balanced in your reactions to others.
Muscles	Our ability to move.
Music	Beautiful music suggests the peace and harmony you find in life. Disharmony is a warning to begin or get back to soothing, spiritual practices.
Mussels	It is important to settle down and thrive through your attachments in love, friendship, and work.
Myna Bird	It's time to speak up. Voice your own opinion as well as focus on positive ways to communicate.
Nails	Protection of self.
Naked	Feeling exposed and vulnerable, or feeling free (depending on the feeling you have within dream or imagery).
Neck	Seeing all sides to a situation; flexibility.
Necklace	Neck = communication; worn near heart = what we treasure.
Nerves	Receptiveness, communication.
Nightingale	Love, emotions, and your expressions of love. Sharing creatively through the written word. Knowing that it is more important that people love you for who you are than how you look or the material possessions you own.
Nine	Number of completion. Handling challenges gracefully. Sharing wisdom with others. Spiritual growth and attainment of principles.
North	Certainty, truth. The direction by which all others are calculated. Introspection, exploration, and responsibility.
Nose	Self-recognition and primitive sensor.
Nursing Child	Nourishing your ideals and goals.
Oak Tree	Strong, durable, resilient. Able to thrive through changing environments and periods of hardship.
Ocean	Womb, Mother Sea, emotions, subconscious mind. The movement or stillness of the ocean will reflect your feelings.
Octopus	It is time to take care of yourself outside work. Clear and clean your environment. Use your intelligence to succeed and thrive in balance.
Olive Tree	Peace through character, tenacity, grace, and sustenance. The olive tree will survive even when cut down or burned. New shoots will emerge from the roots. A message of strength and abundance.
One	The beginning and end, alpha and omega. The primary number from which all others evolved. The oneness of all that is and will ever be.
Onyx	Transform negative energy to build strength and stamina.

Opal	Reflects and strengthens qualities back into the world.
Orange (color)	Energy, cleansing, vibrance, creativity, intimacy, and sexuality.
Orange (fruit)	Health, energy, cleansing, regeneration, and recovery.
Orange Blossom	Hope, energy. Cleansing and healing through aromatherapy.
Orange Tree	Cleansing on all levels, health-centered. Clean up old behavior; utilize new emotional and physical energy for new life.
Oriole	Adaptability to different environments. Monogamy in relationships. A reminder to eat more fruit for your health. There is more joy and sunshine ahead.
Otter	Natural joy and curiosity. Keep your inner child alive by using your creativity. A reawakening of wonderment at life.
Oval Shape	Womb, new beginnings, increase in activity.
Ovaries	Creation and creativity.
Owl	Quiet wisdom, healing powers, feminine energy, seeing and hearing what others might try to hide.
Ox / Oxen	Hard work, laboring with strong determination.
Palm Tree	Flexibility and strength. Weathers great hardships, able to flex and bend through the hardest times and fully enjoy the beauty of the good times.
Pancreas	Sweetness of life.
Panda	Instead of looking at situations as black and white, consider the gray. Do one task at a time, focus, and spend time alone.
Panther	Going beyond what you had ever imagined for yourself. You are stronger from suffering and overcoming. Death, rebirth, magic, and transformation.
Parachute	Taking risks with faith in the positive outcome. Also, feeling saved in some way, possibly at the last moment.
Parakeet	A message of companionship. Are you feeling in need of companionship or having thoughts of leaving a relationship? The message is about new companionship, or someone with whom we should end our association. In ancient Egypt, parakeets represented our own souls.
Parrot	Healing through color and sunlight. Connection with the higher realms. Mimic qualities of those you admire.
Peace Sign	Feeling peaceful or the desire for peace for self and others.
Peacock	Stay grounded while gaining wisdom and vision. Be yourself and allow others to see your true beauty. Reminder to laugh at life.
Pearl	Beauty and self-worth coming from learning to accept irritations. Moving through challenges.
Pelican	Teamwork, buoyancy, releasing heavy emotions, rising above, seeing the lightness of life.

Penguin	Greater awakening through dreams and meditation. Increase of creative and spiritual expression in your life.
Peridot	Healing, good fortune, and strength.
Phoenix	Death and rebirth. Rising above any circumstances. The phoenix is a symbol of renewed strength, power, and resurrection. Something must die to create change for betterment.
Pig	Family protection and fidelity. Rely on your own strength now. Hold true to your standards and be diligent. Move ahead through obstacles with balance.
Pigeon	Shyness, timidity, sacrifice. Do you feel you must sacrifice for love? A message that you are loving, loved, and lovable.
Pine Tree	Healing for lungs and sinuses. Self-love, self-protection, and self-healing creates independence.
Pink	Self-love, self-acceptance, tenderness, and forgiveness.
Pituitary	Control center.
Plains	Freedom, openness, possibilities. New journeys within and new places to venture.
Plane	Rising above the mundane. The ability to move rapidly now, using energy wisely.
Plastic	Pliability, usefulness. Can also refer to "not real."
Platinum	Platinum is a beautiful, shiny, silvery-looking metal used mainly in jewelry. Like silver, it reflects as a mirror. Spiritual illumination.
Playing Games	What type of game are you playing? Is it for fun, skill, or a game that keeps the truth from you or others?
Polar Bear	It is time to learn new ways to move ahead with great strength. A powerful time for learning and becoming what you are meant to be.
Police	Protection, or fear of authority and being accused. Examine in what context you see the police.
Pool	Contained emotions: examine and express your emotions. Can also represent relaxation and recreation if "lounging by the pool."
Poplar Tree	The poplar tree grows very quickly in temperate climates and has a deep root system. The leaves are oval or heart-shaped representing fertility and love. It is famous for its lightweight elasticity, used for many musical instruments.
Porcupine	Focus on enjoying the wonders of life even through life's struggles. Are you letting people's remarks fester within you, or are you using words to hurt others? Lighten up and allow your inner child to focus on wonderment.
Possum	Know when to avert or bring attention to yourself for your best outcome. Examine your ability to adjust behavior when appropriate.
Prairie Dog	Community, sociability, and participation to bring more joy and fulfillment to life.
Praying Mantis	The lesson of stillness. To go within to gather outer power. Use stillness to heal yourself and others. Calm, quiet introspection will assist you to gain peace and power.

Prostate	Masculinity and the masculine principles: action, protection, courage.
Puffin	Abundance, gratefulness, prayer, with a reminder to have fun within spiritual work. Don't take it all so seriously.
Purple	Intuition. Attainment and desire for spiritual wisdom. Royalty and ceremony.
PVC Pipes	Insulation, endurance, and strength.
Pyramid	Mind, body, spirit. Moving upward, ascending from earth (material, secular, divided) to the sky (infinite, unified, spiritual realm). Initiation into higher self.
Python	It is time to be patient. You have a powerful transition occurring now. Be aware of your physical needs. Shed the old, rest and heal.
Quail	Staying connected with social activities is healthy now. Spending time with friends and loved ones will uplift you.
Quartz	Magnification and amplification of spirit. Clearing of the mind for spiritual receptivity.
Rabbit	Fertility, creativity. Pay attention, plan before moving forward, seize opportunities when presented.
Raccoon	Do you feel a need to disguise your true self or feelings, or defend yourself? Use your curiosity and adaptability within your present environment.
Rain	Washing away the old; cleansing and nourishing for new, richer growth.
Rainbow	Beautiful possibilities and hope after the storm.
Ram	Greater mental clarity, creativity, and imagination. Asserting yourself to take full advantage of opportunity now.
Rat	Use any restless energy in a positive way toward a goal. Willingness to adapt to surroundings.
Rattlesnake	Transition. Trust your intuition about others and how you are feeling. Use your increased sensitivity and perception to gain knowledge.
Raven	It is safe to go into the dark to bring forth the light, to gain courage and insight. Be resourceful to manifest your dreams.
Red	Passion, life, survival, power, excitement, intensity. "Stop" as a warning. Anger.
Redwood Tree	Represents rapid growth, adaptability, longevity, and vitality. Striving upwards, while being a harbor to community. Ability for regrowth after harm.
Rhinoceros	Are you forgetting your own gift of wisdom and discounting your choices or opinions? Remember who you are and the innate wisdom you possess. Trust yourself.
Right	As a direction= toward the future, or the "right way" to go. A message to move forward in the most positive way.
Right Side of Body	Represents father, masculinity, active, expressive side.
River	Evolution, time flowing, creation, your life journey. Flow of energy and effort as well as a place and time for rest and renewal.

Roadrunner	You have the energy and drive to get what you want. Balance your home, recreation, and work and plan before you take action. One task at a time, one after the other will get the job done. Take some down time for rejuvenation.
Robin	Freshness, ease, and new growth. Release of opposition or confrontations.
Rock	Unwavering strength, faith, and foundation. Protection and security, i.e. "The Lord is my rock." Rocks can also indicate groundedness, or obstacles on our path, depending on the environment in which they are seen.
Roof	Highest point or ideals.
Rooster	Sexuality, optimism, and directness.
Rose (flower)	Love, romance, and beauty. Note the color of the rose for further meaning.
Rose (quartz)	Love, self-love, healing, and forgiveness.
Ruby	Passion and vitality.
Running From	Fear of something "catching up to you." What are you running from? Are you feeling unsafe, or that you can't keep up the pace in your life at present?
Running Late	Time to organize and focus on what you need to complete for peace of mind.
Sailboat	Making use of all your resources now. Having the power to direct and redirect your route on your journey. Notice the way in which you move over the water: with ease, or difficulty.
Salamander	Rare inspiration for creativity and success. Find the right people and environment to assist you.
Salmon	Trust that you will have what you need to complete your journey. You will be transformed with your healing abilities enhanced.
Sand	Mountains and rocks worn down by time and the elements; the passing of time as well as the impermanence of life and matter.
Sandstorm	Feeling assaulted by life or circumstances. Examine how you react to the sandstorm for more understanding.
Sapphire	Symbolizes value and preciousness.
Scale	Weighing/balancing in decision-making; coming to balance or needing balance in life.
Scarlet (color)	Wealth, power, steadfastness.
School	Where you learn. Education, life lessons. Notice what is happening there, your age, and how you feel about it.
Scorpion	Transformation through periods of solitude, independence, and passion in relationships. Use creative energy for the highest good.
Sea Horse	Providing protection related to a romantic relationship or child. Trust that you are capable of doing so.
Sea Lion	A multitude of creative energy stimulated now. Balance your inner imagination with outer realities for the greatest benefit to you and others.

Sea Turtle	The need to flow with emotions and go within for your answers. You are strong and protective of family and must be in a suitable environment for productivity. Slow down, take time for rest and rejuvenation.
Seagull	Subtle expression assists you to communicate better. Communication between spiritual and secular world. Accent on healthier diet.
Seal	New possibilities and emotional realms are upcoming. Rewards for courage and persistence are coming.
Sequoia (Giant) **Tree**	Ancient wisdom, higher perspectives, wonder, and awe. Growth, adaptability, sanctuary, and protection.
Seven	Representing the spiritual forces of man and nature. Soul development of an individual. A mystical relationship or completion.
Shaking Hands	Time for friendship and connection, or acknowledging and integrating parts of yourself.
Shampoo	Cleansing your thinking. Releasing the old beliefs.
Shark	Your senses and emotions will be heightened. Trust your instincts, keep your eyes on your goal, and act swiftly.
Sheep	Childlike innocence, with the need to conform and belong. Are you too vulnerable, or too untrusting? Look at these aspects of self, and renew faith through community.
Ship	Adventure, journey, exploration of emotions. Take note of the type of ship, persons on it, and the water it travels upon for greater understanding.
Shrimp	Stay grounded. Commune with friends and family to regain balance.
Silver (color)	Elegance, light, reflection, acting as a mirror, spiritual illumination.
Silver (metal)	Precious metal, elegant, graceful, sophisticated, versatile, sleek, modern. Due to reflectability, a mirror of the soul. Spiritual illumination.
Singing	Divine activities, awakening to your own spirit.
Sitting	In between activity and inactivity. Do you need balance between activity and rest?
Six	Divine union, balance of male and female energies. Beauty, symmetry, harmony, as in the six-pointed star (superimposed triangles).
Skating	When we skate, we glide over a floor or ice with ease. It can also refer to "skating on thin ice" or "skating by," meaning skipping details.
Skin	Protection of your inner being, protection from the outside world.
Skull	Danger, death, or questions regarding life and death.
Skunk	Recognize your own abilities and increase your self-esteem and self-respect. You are capable.
Sky	The celestial "heavens," our gift between heaven and earth. Freedom, possibility, change and power. Mother earth and father sky. The sky provides us with calm (blue skies), power (lightning, thunder), rain (clouds), light (sun, moon, starlight), and color/beauty (rainbows)

Slug	Change is positive. Choose your own path. You are capable of creating more than you have thought possible.
Smoke	Transition of matter into spirit, freeing itself, traveling upward. Also, smoke represents spiritual, communal, and cultural rituals and ceremonies. Observe the environment and feeling of where you see and experience the smoke for positive or negative meaning.
Snail	It is time to balance protection and trust within your life. Examine walls you built during childhood. Bring the child out. Learning lessons of discernment.
Snake	Rebirth, renewal, and wisdom. Change and healing; letting go of the old; releasing fear. Transition and ability to absorb much knowledge at this time. Can also denote fear and facing fear depending on the relation/location of the snake you see.
Snow	Purity, innocence, beauty. Coldness, "frozen" emotions.
Solar Plexus	Center of being, center of intuition, self-esteem, and self-confidence.
South	Warmth, strength, health, fire, energy, creativity.
Sparrow	Increasing self-worth and self-dignity to triumph over circumstances. Speaking your truth from the heart.
Spider	The wheel of infinity, the number 8. Spiders weave the web of creation, so delicate and yet strong, between worlds. A powerful reminder that you create your own world. Use written language to inspire others.
Spiral	Journey, path to enlightenment, creation, direction, growth, progress.
Spiral, Fibonacci	Logarithmic spirals, as seen in nautilus shells, flowers, and galaxies that grow in spiral patterns. Akin to the Golden Ratio. The invisible yet organizing, interconnected creator of intelligence.
Spiral (toward right)	Taking the inward out to others (sharing, expressing). Man into spirit. Human striving. Migrating outward.
Spiral (toward left)	Taking the outward in (receiving, learning). Spirit into man. Human receiving. Returning home.
Spleen	Obsession over life and things.
Sponge	Absorbing, receptive, taking in knowledge. Could be a message to remind you to not absorb others issues.
Square	Foundation, stability. Building a strong foundation for yourself. Also, the four elements (fire, earth, air, and water) or four directions (north, south, east, west).
Squid	Be aware of body language, your own and those around you for best understanding. Your ability to read others' moods and motions is becoming acute.
Squirrel	You learn by doing rather than watching. Slow down, ration your energy. Save and prepare for the future. Balance giving and receiving.
Stag	A message to get back to a more traditional family life. Be gentle with yourself and others. An opportunity to express love that will open new doors for you.

Staircase (down)	Moving downward in your life's journey. Traveling to those repressed places within yourself to learn and release.
Staircase (up)	Moving upward in your life's journey. Growing, learning, moving up toward greater wisdom and or spiritual knowledge.
Standing	Being upright, counted, "standing up to" or "for" yourself and your ideals or others.
Star (4-pt.)	Known as the star of Bethlehem, representing spiritual light.
Star (5-pt.)	Man's experiences in the earth through his five senses. Called the pentagram and related to the Golden Ratio.
Star (6-pt.)	Divine union, balance of male and female energies, man's evolution back to God, seen in two triangles, one pointing upward, the other downward. Called the Star of Solomon.
Star (7-pt.)	In the Christian faith, the heptagram or septagram represents the perfection of God and the seven days of creation. In the Kabbalistic tradition, it symbolizes the power of love.
Star (8-pt.)	Recognized by almost all cultures in the world, the octagram is formed by two overlapping squares. It symbolizes balance between the four elements, also balance between yin/yang, positive/negative, masculinity/femininity, and spiritual/material. Also, two sets of four = higher forces or natural laws, such as the law of physics, controlling the lower realms of matter.
Starfish	Follow your own path to your goal. Independence. Using your own innate skills will enable you to reach your dreams. Many possibilities.
Stars	Possibilities, expressing outward, shining your light, using your gifts.
Steel	Strong, durable, tough. Are you needing strength, or is flexibility needed?
Stingray	Stay on track, on purpose. You can trust that the way will unfold before you. You have an ability to see beneath the surface.
Stomach	How you nourish yourself. Digesting life's experiences.
Stone(s)	Calming energy absorbed within a seemingly "inert" material. Stones absorb the warmth or coolness from the environment and act as batteries.
Stork	New birth and understanding emotions. The stork has no voice but communicates well through its specific gestures. Storks are dedicated and protective parents representing caring for the young and the child within you.
Storm	Challenges, conflict, thoughts and emotions brewing.
Stream	A slower pace of the "river of life." A message to slow down; relax and let it flow.
Submarine	Delving beneath, into the subconscious and emotions.
Subway	Using the subconscious mind and intuition to guide you to your destination and desires.
Sun	Yang/masculine energy: action, activity, brightness, passion, happiness.

Sunflower	Focus on brightness, light, and happiness and share it with others. Sunflowers look toward the sun, even through the clouds.
Swallow	Let go of small issues, distance yourself from them and rise above. Stay objective, cleanse your environment to create loving energy.
Swan	Recognizing your own beauty and power. Coming into your own. Expressing self. Ability to understand others with deep perception.
Swimming	Spiritual activity. Moving and working through emotions. Examine the water you are swimming in: is it calm or turbulent?
Sword	Masculine symbol of courage, strength, and protection. Can also represent the ability for violence.
Tadpole	Children, fertility, new dreams and desires manifested.
Tail	Communication/balance. Animals' tails create balance. They are also a means of communication with other animals and humans.
Tarantula	Release old behavior patterns you previously relied upon. It is time to create new responses to protect yourself. Pay attention to your needs.
Teeth	The words we choose to speak. Consider the condition of the teeth. Teeth falling out = feeling unable or choosing not to speak.
Ten	Completion of numbers and great strength. A completion through the return to the One.
Termite	Utilize group support to achieve your goals. Acknowledge your own growth; don't devalue yourself.
Tern	An abundant, migratory seabird that winters in subtropical and tropical regions. The tern flies long distances and is able to thrive in a wide range of habitats, bringing a message of adapting to whatever environment you are in.
Three	Strength. As illustrated in the Trinity or body, mind, and spirit. One contains the idea, two creates the idea together, and three is the fruit of the partnership.
Throat	Our channel of expression.
Tick	Are your relationships unbalanced? Are others affecting your joy and vitality, or you theirs? Create more joy and vitality within your life.
Tidal Wave	Overwhelming emotions or fear. Address the stresses and emotions you are having with those you trust.
Tiger	Manifesting integrity and power in your own life. Use your strength and passion wisely.
Tiger's Eye	Integrating spiritual and material; bringing the divine into reality with integrity.
Tin	A supportive metal to prevent corrosion. Tin is also malleable and transformative. It can be highly polished, meaning self-reflection is important now.
Titanium	Strong as steel, yet less dense. Non-corrosive and resistant to seawater. A message that strength and lightness can coexist. Work with your emotions and the subconscious mind for greater strength.

Toad	You may have to attend to things you do not wish to take care of now. Tend to details, communicate clearly, and you will be rewarded. Living in the emotional world while staying grounded.
Toes	Direction and details moving forward. Left foot/toes = mother. Right foot/toes = father.
Tongue	Be aware of the words and language you use to communicate.
Tool	What is the purpose of the tool? Scissors = cutting. Ruler = measurement of length. Compass = directional assistance.
Topaz	Intuition, courage, and creative expression. In Ancient Egypt, topaz was associated with Ra the Sun God, bringer of life.
Tornado	Feeling out of control within yourself or within your environment. Make small changes each day to regain your sense of control and balance.
Tortoise (desert)	Use your ability to adapt and use available resources now. You might feel you are being tested. Know that Mother Earth will provide all you need. You are a self-sufficient survivor and protector of the land.
Toucan	A desire to be seen and heard. Now is the time to express your authentic self. Use color for healing.
Train	Journey on a prepared route (tracks). Are you on the right track, prepared for your destination? Examine the motion of the train: is it moving forward, is it stopped, or are you missing the train? Community travel, on one route.
Tree	Growth, and the state of your spiritual and physical being. Is the tree nourished and healthy, or weakened? Consider the qualities of the particular tree.
Triangle (to bottom)	Woman, womb, new beginnings, receiving, yin. Taking from the immaterial and creating outward into the world (material).
Triangle (to top)	Man, from earth to God, upwards, action, yang. Man's striving for spiritual wisdom. Moving upward from material to immaterial.
Tuna Fish	You now have the energy and power to act swiftly to get what you desire. Use mental and emotional agility to achieve your goals.
Turkey	Blessings and bounty. Utilize what is around you. Strength in sharing and community.
Turquoise (color)	Water, coolness, calmness, beauty, flow of emotions.
Turquoise (stone)	Spirituality through truth, wisdom, and stability.
Turtle	Motherhood, protection, longevity, groundedness, practicality.
Twelve	Represents the end of one experience and the beginning of another. A combination of forces that bring strength into the world to spiritually replenish it, e.g. the twelve disciples, twelve signs of the zodiac, twelve months, twelve tribes of Israel.
Umbrella	Protection from weather, or changing situations (sun or rain).

Unicorn	Legendary animal of magical and benevolent powers. Reminder to believe that all is possible. Transmuting and manifesting your ideas and creations from the invisible to the visible. Dreams coming true.
Uterus	Holder of creation, creativity.
Valley	Fertility, new life, a time and place for nurturing creativity and spiritual peace.
Vase	Feminine principle of holding, taking in, and nurturing life.
Vehicle	What type of vehicle is it? Automobile, truck (fire, pick-up, dump, etc.), tractor, etc. Note what the vehicle is designed to do. How is it used, and what does this mean in your life?
Vines/Vineyard	A metaphor for the gift of spiritual growth. As a vine is spiritually nurtured, it can grow and bring forth fruit to be shared. Vine and vineyard metaphors are abundant in the Bible, e.g. "I am the vine, ye are the branches; he that abideth in Me and I in him, the same beareth much fruit; for without Me ye can do nothing; this is My commandment, that ye love one another, even as I have loved you." (John 15:1-5, 12).
Volcano	Volcanic emotions. What do you feel is about to erupt in your life? A message to let emotions out constructively to ease the pressure.
Vulture	Remember that challenges are temporary; there is a greater purpose at work. Use available resources to your advantage.
Wall	Separation from, or boundary between. Notice construction of wall and its condition.
Walnut Tree	Hearty strength. Focus on getting more nutrients into your diet as well as eating smaller meals more often. A reminder to set good boundaries and welcome those who create positive synergy in your life. Walnut trees encourage the small animals of the forest to gather around them, signifying a love of animals.
Walrus	Opportunity now to find hidden treasures, physically and psychically. Sensitive to touch. Trust what you feel, and get together in groups of like minded people.
Wasp	Practicality is important now. Use what you already have to fulfill your dreams. Effort creates success.
Watch	Do you feel you have too little or too much time at present? Can also be a message to "Watch" the ways in which you use your time.
Water	Spirit, subconscious, emotions, fluidity, receptivity. Is water calm, still, fast, or turbulent? Water can be cleansing and refreshing, or murky and ominous. Notice the qualities of the water and in what form you see it. (See river, stream, lake, rain, etc.)
Waterfall	Release of emotion for renewal and freedom.
Waves	Emotional and physical movement and release. You can fear the wave, or ride the wave. "Waves of emotion" are a release just as natural as the waves in the ocean.
Weasel	Suspicion and trust. Trust your senses regarding other people. Examine your life and pursue your goals.
Weeds	Those things we need to "clean up" or remove from our lives.

West	Moving toward enlightenment, closer to the Divine. The Israelites moved westward toward the Promised Land. The Navajo tribe relates the west to death, as did the ancient Egyptians and the Celts.
Whale	Awakening through song and music. Creative inspiration. Add light, color, and wonder to your life.
White	Clarity, connection to your spirituality. Innocence or renewed innocence. Cleansed, cleaned. Consciousness, light.
Willow Tree	Beauty, trust, melancholy. Flexibility, emotionality. A reminder to release your feelings and then move on.
Wind	The movement of mental energy in a direction toward desires and goals. Is the wind calm and directed, or unsettling and turbulent?
Wine	In Christianity the symbol of "the body of Christ." Also, friendship, happiness, or drunkenness. Consider in which context the wine is seen by the person visualizing it.
Window	Like the eyes, the "window" of your soul. How are you looking out at the world and what you see?
Wolf	Time to create new life rituals. Take control of your life with discipline and love. Trust your natural instincts. Share in community.
Wolverine	Persistence. A symbol of the wild. Do not surrender. Use your power and drive in the positive for peace and success.
Woodpecker	Power of analysis and discrimination. Get below the surface. It is safe to follow your own life rhythm now.
Worm	Reworking of past issues. Spend time alone to reexamine what was not working and what you need to release for good. Acknowledging and releasing will refresh your mind and spirit.
Wrist	Flexibility, ease of movement to give and receive.
X Sign	Deleting, ceasing, a "do not" message, stopping or failing.
Yellow	Happiness, mental activity, sunshine, togetherness. Light, energy, optimism.
Yin Yang Symbol	Balance or the desire for balance. Also, balance between the active (yang) and the passive (yin) in the personality.
Zebra	Blend in with the group while maintaining your individuality. Free yourself of black-and-white/all-or-nothing thinking by "seeing the gray." Use mental agility and subtlety rather than force when stating your needs.
Zinc	It is time for growth through healing old wounds.

QUICK REFERENCE - USD

*Note: Not every symbol definition is listed in this quick reference.
Look in the general USD if you do not find what you're looking for.

ANIMALS

Alligator	Alligators are excellent mothers, representing new birth and creation. They thrive in mud, the mixture of earth and water that nourishes growth. Their eyes, high on their heads to see above water, remind us of "higher vision." They also digest very slowly, reminding us to "take in new knowledge slowly as to digest it."
Ape	There is a need for clear, precise communication. Be aware of balancing strength and gentleness.
Bat	Transition, rebirth from within. Release old fears. Promise of a new beginning.
Bear	Going within to awaken inner resources to begin using for betterment in your life. Meditation is beneficial.
Beaver	Planning, building for the future.
Buck	The male deer is a reminder to be actively gentle and forgiving of yourself as you enjoy a return to innocence. The antlers are antennae, representing spiritual connectedness and protection. Pay attention to your thoughts and intuition.
Buffalo	Abundance through staying grounded and following the easiest path. Don't make it harder than it is.
Bull	Power, determination, fertility. Stability without stubbornness. Envelop the female energies within yourself.
Camel	Endurance, adaptability. Though your journey might feel difficult, with positivity and determination you can accomplish anything.
Cat	Self-direction, self-approval, and independence. Going inward, focusing on yourself to attain greater independence through learning new, positive survival skills.
Chicken	Fertility, sexuality, and sacrifice. Remember that you have the power of choice in whom you give to.
Chimpanzee	Important to be social and use the tools available. Reflect on your life and use the opportunities given you.
Cougar	Coming into your own power and asserting with gentleness. Take charge of your life.
Cow	Nourishment, motherhood. Greater self-esteem through self-reflection and self-knowledge.

Coyote	Balancing fun and wisdom for your best life. Need for mental stimulation and close family ties.
Crocodile	Primal strength. Bring feelings to the surface for release. Trust your instincts; take advantage of opportunities. Be mindful of your words.
Deer	Gentleness, innocence, spirituality. Use your senses to understand subtle messages around you. Express gentle love to yourself and others. Forgive yourself.
Dinosaur	What is primitive, ancient, extinct, or out-of-date in your life?
Dog	Loyalty, unconditional love, companionship. Note the qualities of the individual breed of dog.
Donkey	Awaken wisdom. Go with the flow. Release stubbornness and complacency.
Dragon	Mystical message of strength, courage, adventure, and power.
Duck	Ducks live on land and water. A message to handle emotions and stay grounded. Emotional comfort and protection. Self-nurturing.
Eagle	Eagles have amazing vision—ability to see long distances. They are persistent and purposeful toward their goal.
Elephant	Ancient wisdom and power. Spirituality, kindness, and affection. Caring for young, elderly, and the sick.
Elk	Strength, power, stamina, and protection. Need for companionship and group support. Diet affecting energy and strength.
Frog	Coming into your own creative power, learning how to control emotions and the words you choose to share. Living in water (emotions) and being grounded (earth).
Gecko	If you're feeling opposition around you, restore order through your actions as quickly as possible.
Giraffe	Seeing the big picture, looking ahead, being prepared. Neck = communication. Important to communicate your feelings now. Also, it can be a message to utilize both your heart and head.
Goat	Important to stay grounded and balance your journey toward your goals. Plan carefully to move to new heights.
Groundhog	Going deep into your life interests. Explore the mystery of death, dying, and rebirth.
Hedgehog	Feeling the need for protection. Use your curiosity now to learn and share insights with others.
Hippopotamus	Examine and utilize your own artistic and healing powers.
Horse	Heightened sensitivity. Time to awaken to your own power and freedom. Movement is important to de-stress.
Jaguar	Reclaim your power. Become a master over your own instincts. Be patient; don't let the past keep you from accomplishing in the present.
Kangaroo	Keep moving forward. Experience is the best teacher. Disconnect from the past and mature. Progress with balance and stamina.

Koala	You're stronger than you know. Sensitivity and individuality require time alone to cleanse and heal.
Leopard	Having the strength and vitality to overcome old patterns that hold you back. Great leaps are possible.
Lion	Strength, courage and protection. Lions are powerful but choose not to fight uselessly. They roar as a warning; a message to use your voice for assertion, not aggression. The lion's mane is a symbol of health and power. Masculine energy reminds you to take action for your betterment.
Lioness	The lioness is a powerful protector of her cubs and provides for them by hunting. A message to honor your feminine energy: intuition, creativity and your nurturing nature. A reminder to use your power assertively not aggressively.
Lizard	Regeneration, adaptability, and resilience. Making changes in bursts of activity and inactivity.
Monkey	Group socialization is important now. Express yourself clearly and ask questions. Enjoy learning and teaching through positive communication.
Moose	Maternal forces, survival, and protection. Pay attention to your inner world and outer subtleties for greater strength and awareness.
Mule	Mules are unique, aware, and intelligent. They were used for transportation in Ancient Egypt (pre-camel) for their endurance, strength and sure-footedness. They can be less reactive than horses; a message to stay emotionally and physically grounded and stay balanced in your reactions to others.
Mouse	Focus and pay attention to details to attain your dreams. Take care of the small things to attain the bigger things.
Ox/Oxen	Hardworking, laboring with strong determination. Are you working too hard or not enough?
Panda	Instead of looking at situations as black-and-white, consider the gray. Do one task at a time, focus, and spend time alone.
Panther	Going beyond whatever you imagined for yourself. Stronger from suffering and overcoming. Death, rebirth, and transformation.
Polar Bear	Learning new ways to move ahead with great strength. This can be a powerful time for spiritual learning and becoming what you are meant to be.
Porcupine	Focus on enjoying the wonders of life, even through life's struggles. Are you letting people's remarks fester within you, or are you using words to hurt others? Lighten up; allow your inner child to focus on wonderment.
Prairie Dog	Community, social ability, and participation to bring more joy and fulfillment to life.
Rabbit	Fertility and creativity. Pay attention and plan before moving forward. Seize opportunities when presented.
Raccoon	Use your adaptability to make desired transformations. Are you feeling a need to disguise your true self or motives at this time? Protect yourself if needed.

Ram	New beginnings. Use your mental clarity, strength, and perseverance. Assert yourself to take full advantage of opportunity now. Trust your ability to land on your feet.
Rat	If you're restless, use this energy in a positive way—toward a goal. Need willingness to adapt to surroundings.
Rattlesnake	Transition. Trust your intuition about others and how you are feeling. Use your increased sensitivity and perception to gain knowledge.
Rhinoceros	Are you forgetting your gift of wisdom and disconnecting your own choices or opinions? Remember who you are and the innate wisdom you possess. Trust yourself.
Rooster	Sexuality, optimism, humor, and spiritual vigilance.
Sheep	Childlike innocence with a need to conform and belong. Are you too vulnerable or too untrusting? Look at these aspects of self and renew faith through community.
Skunk	It's time to recognize your own abilities and increase your self-esteem and self-respect. You are capable.
Snake	Rebirth, renewal, and wisdom. Change and healing, letting go of the old, releasing fear. Transition and ability to absorb much knowledge at this time.
Squirrel	You learn by doing rather than watching. Slow down, ration your energy. Save and prepare for the future. Balance giving and receiving.
Tiger	Manifesting integrity and power in your own life. Use your strength and passion wisely.
Unicorn	Legendary animal of magical and benevolent powers. Reminder to believe that all is possible. Transmuting and manifesting your ideas and creations from the invisible to visible. Dreams come true.
Wolf	Time to create new life rituals, take control of your life with discipline and love. Trust your natural instincts. Share in community.
Zebra	Blend in with the group while maintaining your individuality. Free yourself of black-and-white, all-or-nothing thinking by "seeing the gray." Use mental agility, subtlety, rather than force when stating your needs.

BIRDS

Bat[10]	Transition, rebirth from within. Releasing old fears. Promise of a new beginning.
Blackbird	Pay attention to nature and your surroundings.
Blue Jay	Develop your innate talents and proper use of power. Keep balance of work and pleasure.
Bluebird	Joy, gentleness, unassuming confidence. Connecting with your authentic self and feeling the joy of self-worth.

10 Though a mammal, also listed under "Birds" for readers' convenience.

Canary	Awaken your own voice. Healing and enlightening others and yourself through experiencing your own feelings.
Chicken	Fertility, sexuality, and sacrifice. Remember that you have the power of choice in whom you give to.
Crow	Create and manifest the magic in your everyday life. Intelligence and adaptability. Others will see your deeds. There is no need to call them to others' attention.
Dove	Peaceful, creative, feminine energy. Mourn the old, and look with hope to the new. Believe in love, abundance, and magic available in the world.
Duck	Ducks live on the land and water. A message to handle emotions and stay grounded. Emotional comfort and protection. Self-nurturing.
Eagle	Eagles have amazing vision—the ability to see long distances. They are persistent and purposeful towards their goal.
Falcon	You might feel like your progress is slow, but you can accelerate your efforts. Through dedication and vision, you will bring your goals to life. Focus on the big picture.
Flamingo	Filtration. Lessons of the heart. Discernment in love and expressions of true feelings.
Goose	Symbol of 8. Infinity, fertility, fidelity.
Hawk	Childhood visions and dreams being realized toward your life purpose. Be open to new ideas and inspirations.
Hummingbird	Finding joy in your life. Believe in miracles and know you can surpass your challenges.
Lark	Larks are one of the few birds that sing while they are flying. A reminder to stay cheerful through your endeavors.
Mockingbird	Finding your purpose, recognizing innate talents and expressing them.
Myna Bird	It's time to speak up. Voice your opinion.
Nightingale	Love, emotions, and your expressions of love. Sharing creatively through the written word. Knowing that it is more important that people love you for who you are, not how you look or your material possessions.
Owl	Quiet wisdom, healing powers, feminine energy. Seeking and hearing what others might try to hide.
Parakeet	A message of companionship. Are you feeling in need of companionship or having thoughts of leaving a relationship? In Ancient Egypt, parakeets represented our own soul.
Parrot	Healing through color and sunlight. Connection with higher realms. Mimic qualities of those you admire.
Peacock	Reminder to laugh at life. Stay grounded while gaining wisdom and vision.
Pelican	Teamwork, buoyancy, releasing heavy emotions, rising above—seeing the lightness of life.
Penguin	Greater awakening through dreams and meditation. Increase of creative and spiritual expressions in your life.

Phoenix	Death and rebirth. Rising above any circumstances. The phoenix is a symbol of renewed strength, power, and resurrection. Something must die to create change for betterment.
Pigeon	Shyness, timidity, sacrifice. Do you feel you must sacrifice for love? A message that you are loving, loved, and lovable.
Quail	Staying connected with social activities is healthy now. Spending time with friends and loved ones will uplift and protect you.
Raven	There is no light without darkness. It is safe to go into the unknown to bring forth the light, to gain courage and insight. Be resourceful to manifest your dreams.
Roadrunner	You have the energy and drive to get what you want. Balance your home, recreation, and work. Plan before you take action. One task at a time, one after the other will get the job done. Take some downtime for rejuvenation.
Robin	Freshness, ease, and new growth. Release of opposition or confrontations.
Rooster	Sexuality, optimism, humor, and spiritual vigilance.
Seagull	Subtle expressions assist you to communicate better. Communications between the spiritual and secular world. Accent on a healthier diet.
Sparrow	Increasing self-worth and self-dignity to triumph over circumstances. Speaking your truth from the heart.
Stork	New birth and understanding emotions. The stork has no voice but communicates well through its gestures. Storks are dedicated and protective parents, representing caring for the young and the child within you.
Swallow	Let go of small issues—distance yourself from them and rise above. Stay objective, cleanse your environment to create loving energy.
Swan	Recognizing your own beauty and power, coming into your own. Expressing self. Ability to understand others with deep perception.
Toucan	The desire to be seen and heard. Now is the time to express your authentic self. Use color for healing.
Turkey	Blessing and bounty. Utilize what is around you. Strength in sharing and community.
Vulture	Remember that challenges are temporary; there is a greater purpose at work. Use available resources to your advantage.
Woodpecker	Power of analysis and discrimination; get below the surface. It is safe to follow your own life rhythm now.

BODY

Ankle	Flexibility to move forward.
Arms	Able to hold and experience life's experiences. Opening up, expressing.

Back	Support (emotional or financial) or lack of it. Upper back: feeling weighed down by life. Mid-back: leftover issues from the past. Lower back: issues of financial support.
Body	Your vehicle in this world. Note its condition, and what stands out to you, and how you feel about it.
Bones	Your beliefs, i.e, "down to the bone."
Breast	Feminine, nourishing, giving, mothering.
Chest	Feelings of love and fear.
Ear	Hearing what is being said.
Elbow	Accepting changes and new experiences.
Eyes	What we see and understand.
Face	What we show to the world. Also, a metaphor for "facing" something. Examine details of the face you see.
Feet	Represent our ability to move forward in life.
Fingers	Indicate the details in life and how we deal with them. Thumb: Intellect and worry. Index: Ego and fear. Middle: Anger and sexuality. Ring: Unions and grief. Little: Family and pretending.
Genitals	Masculine and feminine aspects of self as well as sexuality, or feeling shame within sexuality.
Hair	Our connection to the metaphysical, spiritual world and our thoughts that create physical manifestations.
Hands	Ability to share ourselves and our gifts in life. (To hold and to handle life and those we love.)
Head	Consciousness, intellect, ego. Creation through our thoughts. Connection to the divine.
Heart	Love, relationships, self-love, and security.
Hips	Carry us forward with good balance.
Intestines	Assimilation and absorption of energy.
Jaw	The words you say to others. Notice how you are expressing yourself.
Kidneys	Cleansing of toxins from your body.
Left side/body	Feminine side, receptivity, passivity.
Lips	Secure and worthy in speaking up for oneself.
Liver	Releasing the toxic experiences of life.
Lungs	Ability to breathe in life fully.
Mouth	The nourishment and new experiences you take in, and the words you express to others.
Muscles	Our ability to move.

Neck	Seeing all sides of a situation, flexibility.
Nerves	Receptiveness, communication.
Nose	Self-recognition and primitive sensor.
Ovaries	Creation and creativity.
Pancreas	Sweetness of life.
Pituitary	Control center.
Prostate	Masculinity and the masculine principles: action, protection, courage.
Right side/body	Represents father and the masculine, active, expressive side.
Skin	Protection of your inner being, protection from the outside world.
Skull	Danger, death, or questions regarding life and death.
Spleen	Obsession over life and material things.
Stomach	How you nourish yourself. Ability to digest life's experiences.
Teeth	The words we choose to speak. Consider the condition of the teeth. Teeth falling out = feeling unable or choosing not to speak up.
Throat	Our channel of expression.
Tongue	Be aware of the words and language you use to communicate.
Uterus	Holder of creation, creativity.
Wrist	Flexibility, ease of movement to give and receive.

CHAKRAS

Crown	The seventh chakra (sahasrara): access to higher, universal states of consciousness, connection to all. Direct inner perception without form, pure knowledge. Color: violet or white.
Forehead	The sixth chakra (ajna): related to the pineal gland and the nervous system. Access to spiritual wisdom, intuition. Color: indigo.
Throat	The fifth chakra (vishuddha): related to communication, expressing your higher self purely. Color: blue.
Heart	The fourth chakra (anahata): related to the heart, being balanced, open, pure, expansive. Color: green.
Solar Plexus	The third chakra (manipura): related to digestion, elimination, adrenal function, willpower, energy. Color: yellow.
Stomach	The second chakra (svadhisthana): related to partnerships, creativity, sexuality, choice. Color: orange.

Base of Spine — The first chakra (muladhara): also called the root chakra, related to safety, security, balance. Color: red.

COLORS

Black — Mystery, depth, the unknown. Transformation through death, rebirth and introspection.

Black and White — The division of the Whole; for creation and cooperation. Duality: yin and yang, night and day, sun and moon. Also can be: "black-and-white/all-or-nothing thinking."

Blue — Expression, voicing the authentic self, "true blue," peace, tranquility. Sad: feeling blue.

Blue-Green — Using the power of spiritual principles to bring strength to others.

Brown — Earth, foundation. Growth through stability, earnestness, hard work, and practicality.

Dark Blue — Intelligence, knowledge, sincerity, integrity.

Gold — Prosperity, what we treasure, prominence, authority. Grandeur, extravagance.

Gray — Mind (gray matter), balance between black-and-white/all-or-nothing thinking, intelligence, and maturity.

Green — Healing, growth, nature, fertility. Heart, compassion, and hope.

Lavender — Femininity, grace, tenderness, calm, elegance, higher power/purpose.

Indigo — Intuition, spirituality.

Navy — Intelligence, knowledge, sincerity, integrity.

Orange — Energy, cleansing, vibrancy, creativity, intimacy, sexuality.

Pink — Self-love, self-acceptance, tenderness, forgiveness.

Purple — Desiring and attaining spiritual growth. Royalty and ceremony.

Red — Passion, life, survival, power, excitement, and intensity. Can also represent anger.

Scarlet — Wealth, power, steadfastness.

Silver — Elegance, light, reflection—acting as a mirror, spiritual illumination.

Turquoise — Water, coolness, calmness, beauty, flow of emotions.

Violet — Spirituality, purification, creativity, wisdom, and calm.

White — Innocence, purity, lightness. Transformation through spiritual illumination.

Yellow — Happiness, mental activity, sunshine, togetherness. Light, energy, and optimism.

DIRECTIONS

North	Certainty. Truth. The direction by which all others are calculated. Introspection, responsibility, exploration.
South	Warmth, strength, health, fire, energy, creativity.
East	Moving toward the future. Goals, new beginnings.
West	Moving toward enlightenment, toward the Divine. The Israelites moved westward toward the Promised Land; the Navajo tribe relates the west to death, as did the Ancient Egyptians and Celts.

ELEMENTS

Air	Logic and thinking processes. Notice the condition of the air—is it still, breezy, windy? Masculine energy.
Earth	Mother Earth. Wholeness and inclusion of the natural world and all in it. Your own body, your spiritual home.
Fire	Passion. Release/purification. Creation through destruction and transformation. Masculine (active) energy.
Water	Spirit. Subconscious. Emotions. Fluidity, receptivity. Is the water calm, still, fast, or turbulent? Water can be cleansing and refreshing or murky and ominous. Notice the quality of the water and in what form you can see it. (See *Waterscapes*.)

FISH/SEA LIFE

Bass	Balance between masculinity and femininity. If you have many activities going at once, be as fertile as possible and a percentage of the activities will bring forth fruit.
Clam	A message to stay open and truthful in relationships. Examine your part in being open or closed to intimacy.
Crab	Protection and defense. Do you feel you have to isolate? Consider sensitivity and reclusiveness. Is it time to come out of your shell?
Dolphin	Fun, sexuality, energy. Sound and breath healing. Breathe new, fun activities and spirituality into your life.
Eel	Spiritual journeys ahead, of depth and distance. Physical and spiritual growth toward transformation.
Goldfish	Desiring peace and prosperity. Use your intuition in business and work. Create a sacred and peaceful place for yourself to relax.

Jellyfish	By reorganizing, you will succeed. If you're trying to do it alone, begin asking for help. Divide work into smaller tasks.
Koi	Determination and perseverance leading to success. Do not give up. Adapt to your present environment—you will thrive as you practice flexibility.
Lobster	Are you carrying the past with you as protection? Is it time to regenerate and decide how much protection is needed? Lobsters "molt" and release their shells and then regrow them, representing a cycle of regeneration.
Octopus	It is time to take care of yourself outside of work. Clear and clean your environment. Use your intelligence to succeed and thrive in balance.
Otter	Natural joy and curiosity. Keep your inner child alive by using your creativity. A reawakening of wonderment at life.
Porpoise	Intelligent and fast swimmers. They dive to great depths, reminding us to delve beneath the surface for our own answers. They are conscious breathers and must stay awake in order not to drown. Studies show that they sleep with only one half of their brain at a time, so they can swim, breathe consciously, and avoid social contact during rest. This reminds us to protect our rest and be conscious of breathing. Breathwork encouraged.
Salmon	You have what you need to complete your journey. Transformation and healing abilities enhanced.
Seahorse	Providing protection, involving romantic relationship or children. Trust that you are capable of doing so.
Sea Lion	A multitude of creative energy is stimulated now. Balance your inner imagination with outer reality for the greatest benefit to you and others.
Sea Turtle	The need to flow with emotions and go within for your answers. You're strong and protective of family and must be in a suitable environment for productivity. Slow down, take time for rest and rejuvenation.
Seal	New possibilities and emotional realms are upcoming. Rewards for courage and persistence.
Shark	Heightening of senses and emotions. Trust your instincts, keep your eyes on your goal, and act swiftly.
Shrimp	You may be feeling vulnerable and emotional at this time. Stay grounded; commune with friends and family to regain balance.
Sponge	Absorbing, receptive, taking in knowledge. A message to not absorb others' issues.
Starfish	Follow your own path to your goal. Independence. Using your own innate skills will enable you to reach your dreams. Many possibilities.
Stingray	Stay on track, on purpose. You can trust that the way will unfold before you. You have an ability to see beneath the surface.
Walrus	Opportunity now to find hidden treasures, physically and psychically. Sensitivity to touch. Trust what you feel, and get together in groups of like-minded people.

| Whale | Awaken through song and music. Creative inspiration. Add light, color, and wonder to your life. |

FLOWERS

Apple Blossom	Hope, lightness, inspiration.
Begonia	Storing beauty and energy within for the right time to blossom.
Camelia	Love, affection, admiration. Longing for union.
Carnation	Love, luck, and longevity.
Cherry Blossom	Beautiful impermanence. Reminds us that life is beautiful yet fragile. Appreciate the love and beauty all around you, as it is always transforming. Feel safe within change.
Chrysanthemum	Optimism, strength, and joyful heart.
Daffodil	Hope, rejuvenation, new beginnings.
Dahlia	Inner strength, change, dignity. Lasting bond between two people.
Daisy	Innocence, purity, and joy.
Gardenia	Refinement, elegance. Often used for weddings because of their simplicity and sweet fragrance.
Gladiola	Strength and passion.
Hibiscus	Exotic beauty and charm.
Honeysuckle	Enjoy the sweetness and sensuality of life.
Iris	Uniqueness, faithfulness, hope, and wisdom.
Ivy	Strong emotional attachments are a factor. Healthy boundaries are important.
Jasmine	Love, beauty, sensuality, and purity. Healing through the senses.
Lavender	Serenity, healing, relaxation. Soothing sleep for rejuvenation. Good for neurological challenges.
Lemon Blossom	Fidelity, zest, and purification through love.
Lilac	Hope, innocent of love, renewal.
Lily	Humility and the soul's rebirth.
Lily of the Valley	Joy, innocence, and happiness.
Lotus	Preciousness of life, ever-unfolding. Patience to trust life and self, to unfold naturally.
Magnolia	Love of nature, beauty, and sweetness.
Marigold	Associated with the passion and brightness of the sun. Also, the courage and vitality of the lion.

Oleander	A reminder to keep good boundaries and look beyond outer beauty.
Orange Blossom	Hope, energy. Cleansing and healing through aromatherapy.
Poppy	Pleasure, happiness, needing good sleep.
Rose	Love, romance, and keeping secrets. Note the color of the rose for further meaning.
Sunflower	Focus on brightness, light, and happiness and share it with others. Sunflowers look toward the sun, even through the clouds.
Tulip	Deep love, charity, cheerfulness, and perfectionism.
Violet	Virtue, affection, faithfulness, and spirituality.

FOOD

Apple	Knowledge of the duality of life, health, happiness, longevity.
Banana	Energy, fertility, sexuality.
Bread	Sharing, gift of life, the word of God, nourishment.
Carrot	Fertility, health, prosperity, abundance.
Cherry	Feminine aspects, fertility, renewal, purity, impermanence.
Fish	Endurance. From the water element, the depths.
Grapes	Abundance, prosperity, fertility, pleasure, and joy. A symbol of the many gifts of God to humankind.
Olive	The olive tree/branch is a sign of peace or victory.
Orange	Health, energy, cleansing, regeneration, recovery.
Strawberries	Representative of love and passion due to its color and heart shape.
Vegetables	Health, hardiness, strength.

HOUSE: ROOMS

Attic	The higher mind, spirituality. What we have left behind from childhood or later in life. Observe items you see in the attic.
Backyard	What is hidden, not seen.
Basement	Subconscious mind; primal needs and desires. Can also represent those things we wish to not deal with at present. Can be lower sphere of life and choices. Explore the state of the basement.
Bathroom	Cleansing, cleaning, releasing.

Bedroom	Your private life and time. Intimacy, relationships and rejuvenation.
Dining Room	Nurturing, nourishing others.
Kitchen	Nurturing, nourishing yourself; self-care.
Living Room	Represents your life and daily activities. Also, how you live or would like to live.
Roof	Highest ideals.

INSECTS

Ant	Ants work hard as a team. This is the time to use the support of a team while working toward your goals.
Bee	Work, plans, group support and activity. Creating in an organized manner. Enjoying the sweetness and beauty of your success.
Beetle	The beetle (scarab) was revered in Ancient Egypt, as it was associated with resurrection and change. Change is important now, whether moving through it or accepting it.
Butterfly	Transformation. Acknowledge and accept the changes occurring. You are stronger than you think. Look forward to authenticity, joy, and lightness.
Caterpillar	Patience, hard work, surrender, and evolution. Know that all your endeavors will come to fruition.
Cockroach	Adaptability and using available resources. Messenger of cleanliness and cleansing.
Cricket	Rely on your dreams and heightened sensitivity. Trust in what you have always believed. Focus on the positive.
Dragonfly	Attune to the lightness and joy of creativity and change.
Firefly	A hopeful time to realize dreams. Let your light shine and get your creative ideas out into the world. Spiritual gifts are alight. Inspiration put into action can bring great rewards.
Flea	Until changes are made, the irritations you experience will continue.
Fly	Remain stable through unhealthy experiences and environments; they will pass.
Grasshopper	New leaps forward. Trust your instincts. Focus on the new. Grasshoppers only leap up or forward.
Ladybug	You don't need to push too hard for dreams to come true. Allow your desires to manifest in their own time period.
Mosquito	Are you feeling irritated and attacked by others? Take care of unresolved issues to get back to center and feel increased self-worth and confidence.
Moth	Greater physical sensitivity; trust your own senses. Awareness in intimate relationships.
Praying Mantis	The lesson of stillness. Go within to gather power. Use stillness to heal yourself and others. Calm, quiet introspection will assist you to gain peace and power.

Scorpion	Transformation through periods of solitude, independence, and passion in relationships. Use your creative energy for the highest good.
Snail	It is time to balance protection and trust within your life. Examine walls you built during childhood. Bring the child out. Learning lessons of discernment.
Spider	The wheel of infinity, the number 8. Spiders weave the web of creation, so delicate yet strong, between worlds. A powerful reminder that you create your own world. Use written language to inspire others.
Tarantula	Release old behavior patterns you previously relied upon. It's time to create new responses to protect yourself. Pay attention to your needs.
Termite	Use group support to achieve your goals. Acknowledge your own growth; don't devalue yourself.
Tick	Are your relationships unbalanced? Are others affecting your joy and vitality, or you theirs? Focus on yourself; create more joy and vitality within your life.
Wasp	Practicality is important. Use what you already have to fulfill your dreams. Effort creates success.
Worm	Reworking of the past. Spend time alone to reexamine what was not working and what you need to release for good. Acknowledging and releasing will refresh your mind and spirit.

LANDSCAPES

Canyon	Transitional passageway that can protect or trap. Patience, persistent needed to succeed.
Cavern	Deeper, lower levels of the mind. The aspects of self that we sometimes resist and ignore.
Cliff	Suggests change, being on the edge of something new. How do you feel being there?
Desert	Adaptability, using available resources. Working through challenges; purification and initiation.
Forest	Growth, free of constrictions.
Garden	A place of enjoyment and growth in a controlled natural environment.
Meadow	Peace, silence, softness, fertility.
Marsh	Letting go of past emotions and stages of life. Starting anew.
Mountain	Overcoming obstacles. Determination and energy to attain spiritual growth and goals. Communication with higher power.
Landslide	Feeling extreme emotions that need to be released. Feeling unstable. What will bring stability?
Plains	Freedom, openness, possibilities. New journeys within, and new places to venture.

Valley	Fertility, new life; a time and place for nurturing creativity and spirituality.
Volcano	Volcanic emotions. Feelings of anger and frustration held within. Release for new growth.

METALS

Aluminum	Would you benefit from recycling old belongings and opening space for the new?
Carbon Fiber	Know that great strength and flexibility can coexist; malleability is important.
Copper	Earthy, supportive, protective, and nurturing. Energy conductor. Requires balance in energy, as well as in giving and receiving.
Gold	Illuminating the path to success. Represents prosperity, wealth, authority, and glamour. Alchemists considered gold to be the perfect metal, representing the sun. Gold = what you treasure.
Iron	Abundance, masculine energy. Power, growth, strength, protection.
Lead	Toxic metal representing death and transformation. Time to cleanse impurities and imperfections from within.
Mercury	Toxic metal, representing movement, change, fluidity, and mystery. Time to make positive changes.
Metal	Strength, fortitude, tenacity.
Platinum	Platinum is a beautiful, shiny, silvery-looking metal used mainly in jewelry. Like silver, it reflects, as a mirror. Spiritual illumination.
Silver	Precious metal; elegant, graceful, sophisticated. Versatile, sleek, modern. Due to reflectivity, a mirror of the soul; spiritual illumination.
Steel	Steel is a composite, a message that bringing differing aspects or people together creates greater strength. Strong, functional, versatile, durable.
Tin	A supportive metal to prevent corrosion. Malleable, transformative. Self-reflection important.
Titanium	Strong as steel, yet less dense. Noncorrosive and resistant to seawater. A message that strength and lightness can coexist. Work with your emotions and the subconscious mind for greater strength.
Zinc	It is time for growth through healing old wounds.

NUMBERS

One	The beginning and the end. Alpha and Omega. The primary number from which all others evolve. Independence, originality, leadership.

Two	The number of opposites attracting: sun/moon, dark/light. Duality. The beginning of the division of the Whole: creation, cooperation.
Three	Strength. As illustrated in the Trinity, or body, mind, and spirit. One contains the idea, two creates the idea together, and three is the fruit of the partnership.
Four	Symbolizes man in physical form, in the material world. Four also represents the four corners of the earth, north, south, east, and west, as well as the four elements, earth, air, fire, and water. Four is a foundation.
Five	Representing activity and manifestation. Change, into whatever activity with which it is associated. Business and career.
Six	Divine union, balance of masculine and feminine energies. Beauty, symmetry, harmony, as in a six-point star (superimposed triangles). Home, family matters.
Seven	Representing the spiritual forces of humans and nature. Soul development of an individual. A mystic relationship or completion.
Eight	Creating abundance through confidently using the talents you were given. Balancing work with spiritual principles to support self and others.
Nine	Nearing completion. Handling challenges gracefully. Sharing wisdom with others. Spiritual growth and attainment of principles.
Ten	Completion of numbers and greater strength. A completion through return to the one.
Forty	A period of change, testing, and tribulation, the number is mentioned in the Bible over one hundred times. Forty years was also used to represent one generation or an "epoch."

NUMBERS - ANGEL NUMBERS:

11	The master number, reminding you to listen to your deeper intuitive voice to manifest.
22	Reminder that you can make your dreams into reality. Create.
33	Manifestation and expansion of your desires and talents through your actions.
44	A reminder of self-discipline to accomplish your goals. You have the energy.
55	Changes bringing you to your soul's purpose.
66	A message to remember the divine presence is within you and all around to assist you.
77	You are being congratulated and encouraged as you share inner wisdom through your life purpose.
88	Regarding career, success, financial abundance. Focus on the positive and work toward that.
99	A message to work on realizing your soul's purpose toward helping others.
111	A new beginning, awakening to spirituality, paying attention to thoughts and intuition.

222	Balance and cooperation needed. Patience and diligence to make dreams come true.
333	Joy in creation, manifestation, and completion. You are supported by the angels.
444	Encouraging your determination to lead you to desired goals. Stay on course.
555	Reminder that the changes, hard work, and risks you are going through are worth the benefit.
666	Reminder that spiritual attainment is more important than money and financial attainment.
777	You have the ability to bring hidden spiritual wisdom into creative expression in the world.
888	Opportunities and the ability to bring abundance to yourself and others through your endeavors.
999	Transition is coming in a new mission or higher calling for you. Service through an altruistic venture.
1111	Be mindful as your thoughts manifest easily into reality now, subconscious into spiritual and physical realm.
2222	Have faith; in partnerships, cooperation, peace, and balance. Trust that improvements are possible.
3333	Signifies creativity and spiritual growth. Remain confident, do not be shy of sharing your gifts with the world.
4444	Hard work pays off. Begin or continue to put your ideas into form in the world. You have celestial assistance.
5555	Achieving your goals through shutting out distractions. With focus and optimism, you can make it happen.
6666	Use your imagination and intelligence to balance spiritual and physical work. Balance brings happiness.
7777	Your wishes and dreams are on track. Your hard work and good attitude bring rewards.
8888	Amplified reminder that what comes back to you is what you give out, including financial abundance.
9999	A powerful number reflecting an endeavor near completion. A new start; love to give and receive.

SHAPES

Arrow	Pointing up = toward spirituality, or 'up' in mood or in life. Pointing down = downward, 'feeling down,' decreasing in mood, health, or happiness. Left = past, shadow, feminine qualities, yin, passivity. Right = future, light, masculine qualities, yang, activity.
Circle	Wholeness, inclusion, completion, balance of power, belonging, embracing, infinity.
Circle with Dot	Home, self. Take note of the context in which you see this symbol.
Crescent	Represents the crescent moon, symbolizing yin, receiving, fertility, and silver: reflection, illumination.
Cross	A meeting point, decision, at a crossroad. Symbol of Christ; resurrection.
Diamond	Clarity, wisdom, possibilities.
Dots	A dot is a 'point.' The dot is found in ancient cave paintings. It is a point of time or location. More than one dot becomes relational, and meaningful in its placement.
Heart	Love, relationships, self-love, and security.
Hexagon	Communication, balance, union, and harmony. Home and family; the number six.
Infinity Symbol	The "sideways 8" represents the infinite universe and infinite everlasting time. All that was, is, and will be: Alpha - Omega, eternity.
Lines	Linear ideas manifesting into material. Boundaries, thoughts.
Octagon	Eternal life, infinity, renewal = eight. Used in sacred buildings throughout the world.
Ouroboros	Snake or dragon swallowing its own tail: representing the cycle of rebirth, completion, unification, regeneration, eternity.
Oval	Womb, new beginnings, increase in activity.
Pyramid	Mind, body, spirit. Moving upward, ascending from earth (material, secular, divided) to the sky. Infinite, unified. Spiritual realm. Initiation into higher self.
Rectangle	Foundation, like the square. Stability, trust, honesty.
Spiral, Fibonacci	Logarithmic spiral, as seen in nautilus shells, flowers, and galaxies that grow in spiral patterns. Akin to the Golden Ratio, an invisible yet organizing creator of intelligence.
Spiral, Left	Taking the outward in (receiving, learning). Spirit into man. Returning home.
Spiral, Right	Taking the inward out, to others (sharing, expressing). Man into spirit. Outgoing migrations.
Square	Foundation, stability. Building a strong foundation for yourself. Also, the four elements, fire, earth, air, and water, and the four directions, north, south, east, and west.
Star, Five-Point	Man's experiences in the earth through the five senses. Called the pentagram.

Star, Six-Point	Divine union; balance of male and female energies, man's evolution back to God. Seen in two triangles, one pointing upward, the other downward. Called the Star of Solomon.
Star, Seven-Point	In the Christian faith the heptagram or septagram represents the perfection of God and the seven days of creation. In Kabbalistic tradition, it symbolizes the power of love.
Star, Eight-Point	Recognized by almost all cultures in the world. The octagram is formed by two overlapping squares: symbolizing balance between the four elements, yin/yang, positive/negative, masculinity/femininity, and spiritual/material. Also, two sets of four = higher forces; natural laws such as the laws of physics, control the lower realms of matter.
Star	Possibility, expressing outward, shining your light.
Triangle	Trinity: Father, Son, Holy Ghost; time: present, past, future; humans: mind, body, spirit
Triangle/Circle	AA symbol with the triangle representing the three-part answer: unity, recovery, service. Physical, mental, spiritual, with the circle representing wholeness, oneness.
Triangle, Down	Femininity, womb, new beginnings, receiving, yin. Taking from the immaterial, and creating outward into the world, to become material.
Triangle, Up	Masculinity, upward from earth to God. Action, yang. Striving for spiritual wisdom; moving upward from material to immaterial.

STONES/GEMS

Agate	Stability and grace.
Amber	Going within for ancient wisdom and healing. Warmth and empowerment.
Amethyst	Peace, beauty, and healing of wounds through intuition and spirituality. Prayer and protection.
Aquamarine	Peace, tranquility, balance. Truth in communication and emotions.
Citron	Strength, attracting financial abundance and success.
Diamond	Clarity and wholeness. A diamond ring indicates relationships, love, and commitment. Consider aspects of the diamond (color, shape, size).
Emerald	Healing and balancing the heart. Growth, rest, and rejuvenation.
Garnet	Stone of strength, healing, and spiritual regeneration.
Gold	Illuminating the path to success. Pay attention to what you treasure. Gold also represents prosperity, wealth, authority, and glamour.
Granite	Strength, endurance, beauty, and diversity.
Lapis Lazuli	Connecting to higher power, wisdom, spirituality, to communicate into the world.

Onyx	Transform negative energy to build strength and stamina.
Opal	Reflects and strengthens qualities back into the world.
Pearl	Beauty and self-worth coming from learning to accept irritations; moving through challenges.
Peridot	Healing. Good fortune and strength.
Quartz	Magnification and amplification of spirit. Clearing of the mind for spiritual receptivity.
Rock	Unwavering strength, faith, and foundation. Protection and security, i.e. "The Lord is my rock." Rocks also can indicate groundedness, or obstacles in our path, depending upon the environment in which they are seen.
Rose Quartz	Love, self-love. Healing and forgiveness.
Ruby	Passion and vitality.
Sapphire	Symbolizes value and preciousness.
Silver	Elegance, grace, sophistication. Versatile, sleek, modern. Due to reflectivity, a mirror of the soul.
Stone	Calming energy absorbed within a seemingly 'inert' material. Stones absorb the warmth or coolness from the environment and act as batteries.
Tiger's Eye	Integrating spiritual and material, bringing the divine into reality with integrity.
Topaz	Intuition, courage, and creative expression. In Ancient Egypt, topaz was associated with Ra the Sun God, bringer of life.
Turquoise	Spirituality, through truth and wisdom.

TREES

Apple	Love, health, affection. Family life and generosity are important.
Acacia	Adaptability and endurance. Learning and resurrecting from tumultuous times.
Ash	Strong, ambitious. Functional, useful and needed. Use your talents and praise others to be praised yourself.
Aspen	Transformation and strength through community, communication, and cooperation.
Bamboo 'Tree'	Bamboo is actually a grass, but can be treelike in appearance and stature. It is resilient and flexible while still strong and durable. Stress applied to bamboo, as opposed to wood, is evenly distributed over its surface, reminding us that we can stay balanced and resilient under stress.
Banyan	Groundedness, endurance. Stay grounded and create positive boundaries with others.
Baobab	Survivor. Being positive and using the resources you have at hand allows you to thrive.
Beech	Depth, culture, and physical activity.

Birch	Love of nature and calm environment. Healing qualities; needs to share.
Cedar	Strength, endurance. Healing, purifying and fragrant. Used in spiritual prayer.
Cherry	Beautiful and impermanent. Reminds us that life is beautiful yet fragile. Appreciate the love and beauty all around you, as it is always in transition. Feel safe within change.
Chestnut	Healing properties. Balance of feminine (yin) and masculine (yang) qualities. Bring desires into the outer world and act on them to succeed. A reminder to eat a more natural diet.
Cypress	Strong, sensitive, and empathic. Healing qualities. Capable of dealing with others' emotions well. Reminder to not get bogged down by others' feelings.
Elm	Are you being tough on yourself or others? Release superficial concerns, and focus on a deeper connection with yourself.
Eucalyptus	Strength, survival, healing, and protection.
Fig	Use this time for growth, to open up and communicate, creating greater peace.
Hazelnut	Groundedness. Creating a nurturing environment for others. Love and companionship is very important.
Joshua Tree	Patience, independence, growth. The Joshua tree waits years for its own maturity to begin flowering. Once it flowers, it must grow in an entirely different direction. This suggests that the energy and change needed for new endeavors are available to you by changing your thinking and direction.
Laurel	Nobility, victory, truth, and honor. Self-moderation and balance.
Lime	Warm, exotic climates for health. Adaptability and ability to turn negative situations into positive. A healthy diet to cleanse and de-stress.
Magnolia	Beauty, endurance, sweetness of life. Creating beauty from your interior life (yin) and sharing it with the world.
Mango	Prosperity, fertility, and variety. Mangoes are also very healthy; their leaves have antioxidant and antimicrobial properties.
Maple	Independent, distinctive, original. Sometimes the center of attention. Brings lightness and joy. Hardworking, functional, and nurturing.
Oak	Strong, durable, resilient. Patience needed. Capable of going through periods of hardship using reserve of depth of spirit. Able to thrive through changing environments.
Olive	Peace through character, tenacity, grace, and sustenance. The olive tree will survive even when cut down or burned. New shoots emerge from the roots, maintaining the tree's strength and ability to bear fruit.
Orange	A message to take care of your health. Trust your intuition and cleanse yourself on all levels. Clean up old behavior; utilize new emotional and physical energy for new life.
Palm	Flexibility and strength. You are able to weather great hardships, have an active imagination, and love to help others. Ability to flex and bend through the hardest times and fully enjoy the beauty and adventure of the good times.

Pine	Self-protection and self-healing create independence. Harmony, affection, and reassurance. Creativity with the written word.
Poplar	The poplar tree grows very quickly in temperate climates and has a deep root system. The leaves are heart-shaped, representing love and fertility. It is famous for its lightweight elasticity used for musical instruments.
Redwood	Represents rapid growth, adaptability, longevity, and vitality. Striving upwards, while being a harbor to community. Strong ability of regrowth after harm.
Sequoia	(Giant Sequoia.) Ancient wisdom, higher perspectives, wonder, and awe. Growth, adaptability, sanctuary, and protection.
Walnut	Hardy strength. Focus on getting more nutrients into your diet as well as eating smaller meals more often. A reminder to set good boundaries and welcome those who create positive synergy in your life. Walnut trees encourage the small animals of the forest to gather around them, signifying a love of animals.
Willow	Beauty, trust, and melancholy. Flexibility, emotionality. A reminder to release your feelings and then move on.

WATERSCAPES

Beach	Land (foundation/groundedness) and water (subconscious/emotions). Staying grounded in emotions. Need for relaxation, rejuvenation in nature. Need to look beneath the surface for answers.
Flood	Overwhelmed with emotions, not knowing how to release. Release a bit at a time.
Fountain	Flowing water; spirituality, renewal, beauty, and truth.
Lake	Emotions, contained, receptive, and wise. Feminine energies of absorption, inner power, and passivity. Note conditions of water, still or disturbed.
Ocean	Womb, mother. The subconscious mind. Depth, emotion, fluidity, life. The feminine.
River	Evolution, time flowing, creation, your life journey. Flow of energy and effort as well as a place and time for rest and renewal.
Stream	A slower pace of the "river of life." A message to slow down, relax, and let life flow.
Tidal Wave	Overwhelming emotions or fear. Address the stresses and emotions you are having with someone you trust.
Water	Spirit, subconscious, emotions. Fluidity, receptivity. Is water calm, still, fast, or turbulent? Water can be cleansing and refreshing or murky and ominous. Notice the qualities of the water and in what form you see it.
Waterfall	Release of emotion for renewal and freedom.
Waves	Emotional and physical movement and release. You can fear the wave, or ride the wave. "Waves of emotion" are a release just as natural as the waves in the ocean.

WEATHER

Blue Sky	Fair weather, good conditions, happiness, freedom.
Cloud	Between the seen and unseen. Manifesting your thoughts into reality. Divinity moving into reality.
Drought	Lack of love, care, and nurturing.
Flood	Overwhelmed with emotions, not knowing how to release. Release a bit at a time.
Fog	Inability to see, understand. Confusion, fear, lack of clarity. Wait until it is clear to make a decision.
Hail	A feeling of adversity and punishment. Self-forgiveness needed.
Lightning	Electricity, shock, excitement, surprise.
Rain	Sadness, forgiveness. Release of sadness to nurture new growth and possibilities.
Rainbow	Promise of beauty and possibilities after the storm.
Sandstorm	Feeling assaulted by life or circumstances. Examine how you react to the sandstorm for more understanding.
Smoke	Transition of matter into spirit, freeing itself, traveling upward. Also, smoke represents spiritual, communal, and cultural rituals and ceremonies. Observe the environment and feeling of where you see and experience the smoke for further meaning.
Snow	Innocence, beauty. Coldness, emotions "frozen." Need of emotional release.
Storm	Challenges, conflict, thoughts, and emotions brewing.
Tornado	Feeling out of control within yourself or by the environment you are in. Make small changes each day to regain your sense of control and balance.

www.ingramcontent.com/pod-product-compliance
Ingram Content Group UK Ltd.
Pitfield, Milton Keynes, MK11 3LW, UK
UKHW050650070725
6753UKWH00054B/1596